Appearances

In The Mirror And In The Mind's Eye

A Collection of Interviews with Women
about Appearance and Self-Esteem

by
Marsha Dowd

edited by
Margaret Veach

To: Jonathan
Enjoy!
Marsha

Contents

ACKNOWLEDGEMENTS

My sincerest thanks to:

JILL, for giving me deadlines

STUDS TERKEL, for inspiring me

TRUDY, for listening and affirming

PHIL, for putting up with the angst

MOTHER, for saying, "You can do it!"

SYLVIE, for promoting the final product

PEG, for editing these stories and loving them

COLLEEN, for saying, "Women will talk to you!"

Everyone who told me their story of appearances

Everyone who has read these stories
and offered feedback

Everyone who has offered advice
and support along the way

INTRODUCTION

Raison was three and a half years old. She had come to live with Joanne and her husband two months earlier, and she was still having a difficult time responding consistently to her masters' commands for obedience. As *The Encyclopedia of Dogs* had explained, Dalmations as a breed were slow to mature. Nevertheless, life with Raison needed to be more dependable, so Joanne registered Raison in a two week boarding school. Classes were to begin on Monday.

On Sunday night, after a romp along the hot, humid lakefront, Raison suddenly leapt from the sofa and uncharacteristically began scratching at the door. When Joanne let her out, Raison fled down the outside steps to the narrow strip of grass along the sidewalk and retched until she was stupefied with exhaustion.

When the vet advised keeping her home from "school" on Monday, Joanne figured that Raison knew she was going to school and was having an anxiety attack! However, further examination of Sunday evening's events convinced Joanne that Raison had probably eaten a spoiled piece of fish on the beach before running herself silly.

Raison's sad, funny, ever-so-human experience reminded me of my own bouts of nausea and vomiting that had accompanied my twice-yearly change of schools from third through eighth grade. Joanne and I laughed as we empathized with what we imagined to be poor Raison's reaction to a dreaded new experience. And we began to talk of childhood events that had not only caused us to "toss our cookies" but also affected us in ways that forged who we are, how we see ourselves (both in the mirror and in our minds' eye), and how we feel about ourselves.

How we see ourselves is often vastly different from the way others see us. That discrepancy accounts for many of our personality quirks, not to mention our self-esteem, values, goals, fears, anxieties and preoccupations. Early self-concepts and self-definitions (often imposed on us by parents, siblings and schoolmates) live for a very long time, confusing the issue of who we really are after a lifetime of experiences which should, but often don't, modify our earliest self-image.

How we see ourselves also has a great deal to do with how we embrace the world and other people in it: how we act and interact; whether we get through life by overachieving or underachieving; whom we choose for spouses, significant others and friends. In short, self-image influences much of what makes us who we are. Participation in an image seminar several years ago introduced me to some very personal questions: "How was your self-concept formed? What experiences in your background led to the crystallization of this self-concept? How does your self-concept direct your actions, your life?"

At the time, I thought those were very sensitive, personal questions to be asked to discuss within a group of strangers. Nevertheless, I found the questions so thought-provoking that I decided to do some one-on-one research, with a vague idea for a book. As a professional wardrobe and image consultant, I had found a natural outlet for my own interests in clothing, fabric, color, texture, design, and the psychology of appearances. The subsequent examination of my own life experiences and resultant attitudes, along with the unfolding of several friends' profiles, completely intrigued me. The number of interviews grew to more than 40 as I investigated this subject with any woman who was willing to share her story with me.

The women I interviewed are not famous, successful, or superwomen. They are women of my acquaintance who were willing to talk about themselves and their sense of self. Some are long-time friends, some are new acquaintances, some are women who simply impressed me as having an interesting viewpoint. They represent a wide spectrum of age, family background, ethnicity, lifestyle, and attitude.

My original intention in doing this project was to find out whether other women have had as difficult a time growing into their appearance and sense of themselves as I have had. Or was my experience unusual for some reason?

What I have discovered is that some women's journey to self-acceptance has been as bumpy as my own, in different ways. Some women felt they had always had a naturally strong and healthy self-image. Some women have exchanged a good self-image for bad, or bad for good, based on life experience or professional help. Some women have struggled throughout their lives gaining or losing ground as circumstances unfolded. Some women have approached the issue with thoughtful deliberation throughout their lives and some have given it little or no thought. Some women had much to say in response to each of my questions; others felt hard pressed to answer the questions or to give me what they thought I wanted.

The questionnaire I developed as the outline for each interview was based on chronology, as well as personal outlook and family culture. Family cultures have a profound impact in many areas of self-esteem: appearance, intelligence, education, talent, gender roles, and filial and familial duty. How the family of origin deals with affirmation, personal power, entitlement, deservedness, inhibitions, adventurousness, focus, direction, values, generosity of spirit, and spirituality all imprint the individual with different degrees of self-acceptance, rejection, or ambivalence.

Experiences differed tremendously. In taping these interviews and then transcribing them, I came to realize how diverse family cultures can be. The issue of appearance has been treated in as many different ways as there are interviews in this book. It is difficult to generalize, then, but "in general," the women whose families emphasized education, talent and ability, athletics, ethics, and social skills had an easier time learning to value themselves for something other than appearance.

Even with family support, however, those women faced a difficult task, as women in this country are judged first and foremost on appearance. Even our most accomplished women in business and politics are constantly subjected to criticism of their appearance. Women of the most outstanding ability are compared physically to models, movie stars, cover girls, and beauty queens who are in turn criticized for their poor taste in clothes! Lots of love and support and affirmation for intelligence, character and ability in the family of origin goes a long way toward developing women who can withstand criticism of their skirt length, their legs, or their hairstyle. And they will need that skill, because as soon as women become accomplished and successful enough to be noticed, they will be criticized by both men and women for their appearance.

Studies have shown that children as young as four or five judge their peers on appearance, and children appraised as unattractive or overweight are literally shunned from play groups. During adolescence, appearance is still the number one factor for popularity, acceptance, and membership in the group. Some of us never outgrow the scars inflicted on us in those years of anxious marginality. Many of us never forget being the last one picked for basketball and softball, even if we have other skills that compensate. The truth is they often don't.

For some, those wounds and insecurities take time to heal; for others, the bruises are negligible and easily forgotten. Thank heavens most of us mature to the point that we love and accept for reasons other than appearance! We choose friends and lovers and mates for their personality, generosity, humor, energy, ambition, creativity or stability. And friends and lovers, and mates choose us for the same reasons. In the long run, the Prom King and Queen are not the only ones to establish and maintain relationships.

However, the question still remains: Why is it more difficult for some women to like themselves than it is for others? Why do some beautiful women find it impossible to like themselves? Why do some homely women find themselves eminently worthy of life's blessings? The answer lies in each person's head, heart and mirror. And the strange and wonderful chemistry therein.

There are many theories found in recent "how-to" books on women's self-esteem, and although the theories are explained using personal interviews collected by the authors, few of the interviews are actually published in these books. It was the lack of interviews with a lifetime perspective that led me to collect my own book of stories. These are the kinds of stories that fascinate me, delight me, and make me cry. They make me see life from many different perspectives. They make me see that we all have our job cut out for us: to find ourselves, and to keep finding ourselves again and again over the course of a lifetime.

There are no new, or even old, theories to be expounded and proven with this book. This is simply a book of shared stories from women who have overcome much to find their own tender feelings for themselves; from women who have learned to live with themselves, or to change what they didn't like; from women who have faced many challenges and have discovered that the challenges never end. These stories are fascinating in their simplicity, their complexity, their frustration, and their triumph— but most of all in their commonality. For it is in the sharing of our stories that we women can find our greatest solace, strength, and inspiration. It is in sharing that we learn to go on, to change, to grow, and to love ourselves as well and as gently as we love others.

May you recognize yourself in one or many of these stories. May you realize that you are not alone, that others have come before you and others will come after you. May you find that sharing is our greatest gift to each other.

This project has been a kind of therapy for me. Writing my own story has been a way to gain new perspective on myself. Others' stories were full of surprises. One interviewee enrolled in graduate level psychology courses to better understand herself. Some women found art, some found business, some found family life, some found the single life as a way to explore themselves. Each one found her own path. And that is the lesson contained in these stories. Each one must find her own way. No one can follow another's route to find herself. Whatever I have learned from this book will not necessarily serve you as well. My answers are not your answers but I sincerely hope that you have found some answers of your own. I hope, too, that you will continue to seek the answers you will need for the future.

Enjoy these stories! They are for you.

QUESTIONNAIRE

What is the first memory you have of yourself as a child? Is it as an individual or in relation to someone else? Was it a positive or negative experience?

What other childhood incidents contributed to your growing sense of self-image. Positive or negative? Did you have sensitivities toward any of your physical characteristics or personality traits?

What role did your parents, siblings, or other relatives play in the formation of your self-image? What did they say or do, positively or negatively?

How did you see yourself in the teenage years in high school?

How did you see yourself in young adulthood?

What role did any of the special men and/or women friends play in the formation of your self-image? What did they say or do, positively or negatively?

How do you see yourself now? What changes, if any, have you made in your self-image over the years? Why? How?

At what point in your life did you perceive your appearance as positive, and pleasing to yourself? What words best describe your most positive mental image of yourself?

Do you feel that your looks were at their best at a younger age? Or do you feel that you look better than ever at the present time?

How do you perceive yourself as a whole? Does your appearance rank equally with your intellect, personality, and achievement? Is there a gap between your mirror-image and self-image?

How do you think other's perceive you? What have others said about you, or not said about you? What have they complimented or failed to compliment? Is there a gap between your own self-image, and others' perception of you as a whole person?

Are you happy with the person you are today? Where would you like to make changes, if any, in the future?

How do you plan to deal with the aging process?

A L I C E, 47:
free-lance interior designer

I have been very tall all my life, but I became especially aware of it in high school. It got me a lot of attention—mostly good attention. Later I discovered that being the tallest in terms of the boy-girl thing worked out well, too, because it got me a lot of attention from short guys! I am probably one of the few super tall women who feels that my height—six feet—has been an asset.

I don't remember problems with my general appearance. Intermittently there were things like wanting to get my teeth straightened or having to wear glasses. There was a time when I thought I had the world's biggest feet! I also thought I had very large, very masculine, very ugly hands, but once I grew long fingernails and learned to do my own manicures, that ceased to be a problem. My favorite relative, Aunt Kate, brought me boxes of her old, out-of-style costume jewelry to play with when I was a kid; she taught me how to care for my hands and inspired me to wear big rings and bracelets.

My appearance wasn't really a positive or negative thing. I remember it more as an issue of having what was "in," like the right little flip hairdo. If it rained on the way to school and my flip fell, I was ruined for life! But that wasn't really an appearance issue or even a hair issue.

I never thought I was good-looking, but I always thought my appearance was good enough. That's why I liked being tall. The only thing that was different about me was my height; if I had been 5' 3", nobody would have looked at me twice! I've always worn high heels to play up my height as my biggest asset. I have heard that French women play up their most unique feature, even if it's unattractive, for the sake of individuality. What a great idea! I've always gotten so much attention for my height, that I never noticed if anyone thought I was nice-looking.

If there was one thing I could have changed, I would have given up being flat-chested. But it has not affected my life very much. Back in school, in gym class, my flat chest might draw a comment from some of the girls—but there were always other girls who were flat-chested, too. Once I got to early middle age and decided I didn't need to wear a bra, I was a liberated woman. I don't wear bras anymore. I never really needed a bra in my entire life. And all those years I wore them so tight just to hold them in place! I went around with heartburn all of my twenties because of tight bras. Now I am glad I don't have a chest because it's more comfortable and I don't have to worry about droop.

Good posture was a big part of my upbringing, thanks to my grandmother. I walked with books on my head and got knocked around if she caught me slumping. It was very important to stand up tall and proud as a good Southern woman.

My grandmother had a very positive effect on the formation of my self-image. The two most important rules were: stand up tall and proud, and be clean. Rule number three was "be ladylike." If I did something that wasn't ladylike, I'd get my mouth washed out with soap or get switched with a branch of forsythia! I also knew that if Granny caught me with my knees apart, I was going to get it. And if I really did something bad it was the hairbrush on my bare bottom. My grandmother's old-timey bone hairbrush and mirror set had an elaborate P carved in it. When she got through with me with that hairbrush, I had perfect Ps all over my butt! I always thought that was so neat. I would go look in the mirror to see all those Ps. My grandmother got me through my whole life with never a concern about how I looked. Her emphasis on manners and posture made physical appearance irrelevant. That mastery of situations made me very self-confident in any social situation.

I have always had a positive mental image. I used to have days when I knew I looked like a million dollars and even felt especially tall. It's important to know that I can make people believe something that is all illusion. For instance, people have always told me what good legs I have.

And I do not have good legs! I have very long legs, but I do not have really good legs. I have always had thick thighs and chunky knees. But with the right hose, very high heels, and sitting right like Granny taught me, I can have people believing I have the greatest legs. Just like Marlene Dietrich! I have always thought that was fun, to get attention for great legs.

There was only one time when I didn't feel good about my looks. That was when I first moved to New York to work. I was like a kid in a candy store. I had never had so much good food and drink and bread and real butter. And breakfast, lunch and dinner in restaurants because I was in sales. I got so fat; in six months I put on thirty pounds. And my couple of size sixteen outfits were tight! Then I did not like the way I looked. I felt very negative and I didn't feel good physically. So I dieted and took off the weight and then everything was fine again.

But several years ago, the combination of middle age and quitting smoking caused me to gain back all that weight. I felt really yucky about my appearance, and I realized I will have to diet the rest of my life. I'm not going to worry about aging, but I am going to have to worry about my weight.

Then I hit middle age a couple of weeks ago Tuesday. I was just commenting on how well preserved I was for my age, and four days later, it all fell off! My elbows collapsed, and my thighs fell down around my ankles! When I put on a facial mask, I put it on all the way down my chest; next week I try it on my thighs. Or I just won't look in the mirror anymore!

I looked pretty good as a young person, and I don't think I look bad for a middle-aged old bat! Two weeks ago, I couldn't have said this but I have calmed down now. I see myself now as looking my age—no less, no more.

When I had my teeth cosmetically enhanced two years ago, the new bottom teeth didn't faze me much. But the first couple weeks after the top teeth were done, I was very self-conscious because they changed my facial structure somewhat. I had to learn to smile without grimacing. I smile more often and more naturally now, but I had to actually stand in front of the mirror and practice smiling. I had never really smiled all-out like that before, because of my teeth; I was always covering up braces or bad spaces or, in recent years, eight different colors of teeth from all the root canals. So the first couple weeks after the enhancement were traumatic in a positive way. I wasn't aware of how bad my teeth were until they got so good! However, the dental enhancement has not really changed my mental image of myself!

Although I spend two hours doing my toilette in the morning, I don't primp during the day. I wouldn't think of going to the Dumpster without my full makeup in the morning, but then I walk around all day without replacing my lipstick! Crazy! Of course I have to get started in the middle of the night to be somewhere by 7 a.m.

Recently I learned that the famous Hollywood makeup artist, George, was coming to a local salon for a week. Well, this conjured up fantasies of my youth and the glamour that he represented. He made Linda Bird Johnson gorgeous, just think what he could do for me! The picture of him in the ad was very appealing, so I fell for it and made myself an appointment. As it turned out he had put on a lot of weight, had probably seen a lot of late nights, and was pretty much beat up and burned out. When I got to the salon, he was eating Chinese food out of the carton, and telling me my hair was too short. Then he proceeded to put makeup on me that went out of style with Linda Bird Johnson! He put purple on my eyelids. Well, I'll spare the details but it was just gross what this man did to my face! And I have never been as old-looking as I was when I walked out of that salon.

But what I really learned from that incident is to keep up with the times. I have actually been doing a great job; old George hasn't kept up as well as I have. So I am still going to keep frequenting makeup artists, and I am still going to keep playing with makeup, but I am not going to any more has-beens. I want today's new modern miracle-maker and the magic of subtlety! And the moment they pull out purple, I'm heading for the front door! My vanity cost me only $350, but I learned my lesson.

Apparently, a lot of people are intimidated by me, and I have always thought that was very strange. People have said that when they first met me they found me very intimidating. I don't understand that—except for my size. Finally a friend passed on some of her perceptions of me. She says it has to do with my body language, my comfort level with my height, my wardrobe, personal style, and also my manners—all that stuff that my grandmother whipped into me. According to my friend, Northerners don't act like I do, so it's almost as if I am from a different country! There is a different culture in the South than there is in the North. But other than that, how others perceive me I really don't know. I have often wondered.

I am happy with the person I am today, but that happened only yesterday. I think that having no plans and no goals is a real rip! For the first time in my life, I am going nowhere and I rather like it! The most important thing in my life these days is, what's for dinner? Or lunch or breakfast? Coffee break or cocktail hour! I harbor the idea that I may stumble over something overwhelming to visit, or see, or be, or learn, or study. But the way I feel today, if I don't, that's also fine. I am determined to age like Katharine Hepburn. Get me some of those pants and shirts and just "chill out," as the kids say.

A NITA, 29:
hairdresser

My first memories of my appearance are from pictures of me looking like a brunette Bozo with my thick, curly and unruly hair. My younger sister was the "pretty one," with dark skin, green eyes, and shiny, black, long, straight, beautiful hair. Although everyone in my family is small, she was extremely petite and designated the best-looking. I don't think the comparison was a completely negative experience for me or I wouldn't be who I am today. And it has changed over the years—ultimately she didn't remain the prettiest.

My pivotal childhood memory is this: In my preteen years, my dad went to a fortune teller, a card reader who had been recommended to him. This woman told him that one of his three daughters was going to give him problems. Two of his daughters were going to be fine; they would marry and have children. But the problems were just beginning with his third daughter. She warned him to be prepared.

When my dad came home, he sat me down, and with tears in his eyes, told me that I was supposed to be that troublesome daughter. He wanted to warn me so I wouldn't turn out that way. Of course, that was a very negative thing to say; nevertheless, it turned out to be quite positive because I felt I had a lot to prove to my dad, and slowly but surely I did! I mentioned this incident to him about four months ago and he said he still remembers the conversation but he didn't take it seriously. I looked him straight in the eye and said, "I will never, ever forget and I am still trying to prove you wrong!"

I am the most sensitive in my family. I think that comes from being the middle child and having to act differently than my sisters to get attention. If I hadn't acted sensitively or emotionally, my family wouldn't have paid any attention to me. So if I cried, I always exaggerated to get a little more attention. Then they called me a crybaby because I cried for anything and everything. I am still sensitive; if someone raises their voice to me, I get upset.

My parents are Puerto Rican. My dad came to work in the United States; my mom was brought here by her stepmother. My mom and dad met, lived together, and had three children before they got married, which was scandalous in those days. I am the middle child of three—Yolanda, myself, and Sylvia.

My oldest sister Yolanda had her daughter Sophie when she was 21 and lived with her boyfriend for ten years before they got married. My sister Sylvia has a daughter, Giselle, and is not married; she says she will never marry! I lived with my husband for a year before I got married at age 26, but I didn't have any children before marriage.

Mom was never one to care about how she looked while we were growing up, so we were not taught to care about appearances. When we got into our preteen years, our Aunt Nellie took over. At that stage she bought us makeup, taught us how to shave, tweeze our eyebrows, and blow-dry our hair. She was our fun, cool aunt with three younger daughters of her own. She would say, "This is what I'll teach my daughters to do, so why don't you girls do it too. Let's try this, let's do that!" My mom's opinion was, "Oh my goodness, take off that makeup. Take down that hair. You look like a plucked chicken with all your hair shaved and your eyebrows gone!" She was never one to compliment anything that we did for appearance's sake.

I went to public high school on the southwest side of Chicago. It was 75 percent black and 25 percent Hispanic. I started as an honor student my freshman year. But near the end of my first year, I started hanging around with several other girls who were cutting classes. No more honor roll. During my sophomore year, some of these friends started getting out of school early to attend beauty school. "We leave the high school at twelve o'clock, and take the bus to the beauty school starting at one o'clock. But we don't really go to beauty school, we go to the beach, and the museum, and we hang out!" It was a special program which only bilingual students could join. And it cost only $100.

I went home and begged and cried exaggeratedly for $100. My father refused because it was a three-year program, which would preclude my going to the commercial business school downtown. There was no way he was going to let me become a plain old beautician instead of getting a good business school education like my older sister. At the commercial school, students wore hats and gloves and makeup and looked professional; they were trained for the business world.

But after begging and crying for months, I finally broke through my dad's defenses and joined the beauty school. In my last year, I started getting serious; my teachers started paying attention to me and I really liked what I was doing. I didn't think I'd like it so much, but everything really came together that last year. At the end of the three years, I graduated from beauty school at the same time I got my high school diploma.

High school flew by. Every minute was fun. In my senior year I was prom queen, homecoming queen, and was voted best personality. But I didn't have a date until the day before the prom because nobody thought to ask me. I was just too popular! My prom date, Romeo, was the date from hell, but the year made up for it in other ways.

I lived in one gang's neighborhood and went to school in a rival gang's neighborhood, but because I was so sociable, nobody ever bothered me. It wasn't Disneyland, however. Many house parties during those years ended in shots fired and everyone scattering. Many times I was frisked by the police for loitering in the neighborhood of my high school. It eventually became a closed campus because too many students were injured outside the grounds when rival gang members drove by and shot from their cars. Many times I ran into a gangway to hide or into a total stranger's house because shots were being fired.

I saw my niece's father get shot in the leg for no reason when a young kid who was showing off with a gun across the street from the school playground fired it by accident. During the four years of high school, five of my friends were killed by rival gangs. A neighbor of ours was hiding a gun in his bedroom when his younger brother found it and, showing off to his best friend, accidentally fired it. He shot his best friend in the head and killed him.

My father insisted on meeting all our friends so that if neighbors or family commented, he could say, "Oh I know him, he's a nice guy." So my father knew all our gang-banging friends and he would sit them down and preach to them. But he wouldn't say, "Give me the gun." He would just say, "Do you know what you're doing? Do you want to be alive in ten years? Stop doing that."

Sylvia and I were part of a "gang" of about fifteen girls—a dancing gang, not a killing gang. We called ourselves The Girls. There was also The Boys group. Every weekend we showed off: someone in the group had a house party where we danced or we went out someplace to dance. During the week we practiced, so, of course, everyone knew how to dance with everyone else, although certain people danced better with certain partners. I entered three major dance contests with my partner. We got second place in one and first place in another!

I realized that I was cute at the age of 13. The whole world changed when I turned 13; I got my period and became a woman. And then my father let me do things that a woman could do, dress and act more mature, cut and straighten my hair. I had plucked my eyebrows even before my dad agreed to let me wear eye shadow and eyeliner, but he wouldn't let me wear lipstick until later.

And I could go shopping! When North Riverside Mall opened, my father got his first Mastercharge, which he let us use. That was when I discovered clothes and my own style. Until we turned 13 my mother bought everything we wore, but as soon as I turned 13, my sister Yolanda got the car and my father's charge card and we went shopping. So, little by little, I started coming out of my ugly closet.

For me, young adulthood started at the age of 17 when I graduated simultaneously from high school and beauty school and got my first job. And in my family, along with your first job, you proved yourself by becoming responsible for one of the household bills. My responsibility was the gas bill, but every penny I had left after that was mine to spend. That's when I became a responsible person: saving money for a car, my own clothes, my own charge accounts.

When my older sister graduated from high school my dad gave her a Visa card. She charged to the limit and gave it back to my dad without paying anything. When it was my turn, I said, "No thank you, I'll get one in a couple of months on my own." He laughed at me, but about six months later I got my own Visa. I was always proving myself to my dad. I never let him give me anything. With my Visa card I was really careful; I never ran it up to the limit. I also saved $1,200 to buy my dad's car from him. The fact that I bought it from him—he didn't give it to me—reflects really well on me.

As a young adult, I could have made many mistakes. But being the responsible type and wanting to prove so many things to myself and my parents, I didn't allow myself to get into situations that could have been dangerous. As far as sex and pregnancy goes, the opportunity was there but I always thought about it and decided against it. So at the age of 18 I got on birth control. Responsible, that's me.

Whether I chose them consciously or not, most of the friends I hung around with were large, overweight, or plain people. As a result, I always got the attention because I was the cutest and the most adventuresome. My friends always pushed me to do things that they didn't have the confidence to try. That did a lot for my self-confidence.

It's really hard for me to talk about my self-image without discussing my sister Sylvia. We were born in the same family, to the same parents, only 11 months apart. We shared the same bedroom and the same clothes up until our teenage years. We had exactly the same friends; we sometimes had the same taste in boyfriends. We went everywhere together. But Sylvia was and still is a plain Jane. At 13, when I started wearing makeup and taking care of myself, Sylvia did the complete opposite. She never tweezed her eyebrows, never wore makeup. She cared very little about her looks in any situation, whether professional or personal.

It bothers me so much that lately I have tried to do a little something for Sylvia's appearance every month. She doesn't know how to deal with it. She doesn't want to change or become prettier. She still has her looks, but she just doesn't know how to bring them out in any way. Finally, when it became a professional issue related to raises and promotions, she began to get the idea. So Sylvia has changed somewhat for work but she still doesn't know it's important for her personal life. Most people don't even realize that Sylvia and I are sisters because our self-image is so different.

My first job out of high school was as a neighborhood hairdresser. I was hired sight unseen over the phone because of my beauty school's recommendation. After that I worked in neighborhood beauty salons for five years. At age 23 I got my first job downtown in a haircut factory. Six months later I got the opportunity to work at a corporate image salon and my whole sense of self changed. I went from a neighborhood cool, punky hairdresser to a professional hair designer. From that point I started doing my own hair better, wearing better clothes, making sure that my appearance was conservative. Our look had to be approved by our manager, and that taught me a lot about fitting the part. I was a totally different person at work. On my personal time I would let loose, but when I walked into the salon I was Miss Conservative. And at that point I became more satisfied with my mature appearance and image. I always knew I was cute, but at 23 I became even better-looking with my more conservative image.

I never thought that I was intelligent because I didn't go to business school or get a college education. But I cannot compare a college education with what I have learned from my clients over the years. I think that I carry myself as a very intelligent person. I may be winging it but I can discuss it, whatever it is. Now I want a college education to understand everything about my customers' conversations.

I will never be satisfied with my achievements. There are always more goals. And that's why, at age 29, I am a college freshman. It may not be for a degree, it may only be for myself, for my own knowledge. If I get a degree out of it or if I start my own business, even better. I am not going to set specific goals right now because I don't want to put that much pressure on myself.

I am the most ambitious person in my family. And it all comes from my dad telling me I was the designated troublemaker. That incident has driven me to ambition. Now I want to achieve certain things at certain times in my life and I am really hard on myself until I get there. So far I have reached every goal, even if a little shy of the time limit.

In my mid-20s I planned to move out of my parent's house and into an apartment with my sister Sylvia. In the process of that move, I met my future husband, Rick. Because we didn't have our phone installed yet, he gave me a quarter along with his number and asked me to call him. I promptly misplaced the quarter and the number in the chaos of the new apartment. After some additional pandemonium I found it and called him. That was day one and we haven't been apart since! We moved in together after a year. A year later we got married. A year after that we bought a house. And now we are expecting our first child.

I don't plan on dealing with the aging process very well at all. My philosophy about aging is, if you can improve something, do it. If it costs money, as long as you are not taking food from your family, spend it— it's worth every penny. I probably will deal with age changes to my face better than my body. If my body goes, I will pay as much as I possibly can to take care of it. I can camouflage my face enough with makeup and hair-styling. I would probably get a tummy tuck or liposuction before a face-lift. But I don't see myself taking the aging process very well.

People often comment on the fact that I am a perfectionist when it comes to planning my life. I don't like to do things without a plan. If I can't organize it completely, I plan it in stages. And it usually works out exactly so people are surprised that it turns out according to plan. I said I would get married by a certain age; I did. I said I would have children by a certain age; I have. I am starting my family now and I plan on having two children. People notice that things usually fall into place in my life and they compliment me. Other people say, "I couldn't live like that." And my answer to them is, "I couldn't live any other way."

The second thing people comment on is my personality! I am being honest when I say my personality radiates out my ears. My body is too small to hold my personality! The comments from strangers or new acquaintances are the ones I like the best, because even though they don't know me well, they still comment positively. I have always been very pleased with my personality; I am very happy with the person I am today.

A N N E, 58:
accountant

My baby sister was born on my first birthday. She was generally acknowledged to look like our mother, who was a legendary beauty. Like everyone else in the family except me, she had big round eyes and dark wavy hair. On the other hand, I was told that I looked like our father except for the color and texture of my straight, limp hair. Although handsome, Dad was over six feet tall and had whiskers; I had a hard time even imagining how I would turn out!

Although my sister had dark hair and I had less striking coloring, we were usually dressed alike. Once, when I was still young enough to be expected to take a nap, we had the Red Dotted Swiss Dress Incident. During naptime, I took a pair of scissors to my hated dress, cutting it into shreds. An enormous amount of commotion ensued when my deed was discovered! But at least I didn't have to wear that dress any more. Probably, too, my naps were more closely monitored.

When we were little, my mother was determined to have us look the way she wanted us to look. One of her requirements was that we wear a bow in our hair. She hired a succession of nursemaids until she found one who, with sheer persistence, made us keep the despised bows in our hair. Mother loved to tell that story. It was her triumph over her "heathen" children!

Gradually my sister and I outgrew all the matching dresses, and my mother worked hard at finding colors that would flatter my different and fairer coloring. She and my grandmother made most of our party dresses, shopping with care for pretty fabrics, and I remember loving them.

In seventh grade I grew tall quickly, overtaking many of my classmates despite the fact that I was a year younger than most of them. My hair was still straight and limp, and now my arms and legs were too long. Compounding the problem was the fact that many of my friends were turning into young ladies; I was being left behind, with a little girl's figure. During that time, we received a big box of handed-down clothing from an older cousin. Everyone was delighted but me. The clothes were of beautiful quality, but all were navy blue or maroon. I hated them, but had to wear them all winter. What an awful year that was! I had seldom paid much attention to my appearance, and when I finally did, it was an unhappy experience. By the end of junior high school I was very used to comparing myself with better-looking people and had accepted these self-imposed comparisons as the natural state of things.

One of my closest friends in high school, a beautiful girl, spent a lot of time and thought on her appearance and always looked lovely. One summer when we were in our early teens, she and I visited a classmate. Our classmate's father commented that my friend looked like a fashion model and I looked as if I had gotten dressed in the closet! This was more or less true; I hadn't reached the point where I thought I should be more than clean and neat.

Then, the summer before high school, my mother found a beauty salon that cut straight hair well, and I got a wonderful haircut. (I still think it's true that when your hair looks good, everything else seems to fall into place.) And I had finally outgrown my cousin's clothes, so I could have things I liked. Suddenly, and much to my amazement, I was also turning into a young lady and the boys were beginning to notice me. Of course, I didn't believe any compliments on my appearance, although I knew I was fortunate not to have the concerns of some of my classmates who had skin and weight problems.

We all spent a great deal of time considering what to wear for which event and were most unhappy when we didn't look like all our friends. There was a lot of telephoning before parties to make sure we were making the right fashion decisions. During this period, I didn't compare myself with my friends or classmates, but with pictures of models in magazines. We all did, I think; it didn't occur to us that they set an impossible standard.

During the week, though, most of my attention was devoted to my classes. I know some of the boys were astonished when I made the honor roll. In those days you were either pretty or smart, not both.

There were lots of parties and lots of fun and the next year I was sent to a girls' boarding school. Uniforms eliminated much of the concern about fashion correctness, but you'd be surprised how creative we were within the allowed limits of the uniforms. We'd pin our collars closed or put a sweater on backward, all in an attempt to develop a sense of style. We also became creative with our hair! The peroxide looked much worse on my roommate, who had dark hair with a new orange streak, but even mine almost brought on apoplexy in my mother, who, when she met the Thanksgiving train, described my hair as "plaid."

My father was less than understanding of this whole process. Although he was quick to compliment me on achievement or appearance, he was not approving of all the time spent in front of the mirror. What he didn't realize until much later was that I was not admiring perfection, but looking for flaws!

During boarding school and college I spent some time trying to develop a sense of style, to find clothes and "looks" that were flattering to me but more interesting than those my mother would have chosen. One success, among many failures, was a black and white paisley corduroy raincoat—it was smashing! And it needed little else to make a complete outfit. One measure of its success was that my mother once asked to borrow it! All too often, though, I bought clothes on the "emergency plan" for a particular event. How very many times I did this before I finally realized that it didn't work! My closet was filled with the most peculiar ensembles, worn once, and never appropriate for another occasion. Even today, I still have to work hard at not shopping for the "quick fix."

My husband, Frank, and I were married when I was 21, and much of my young adulthood was spent in maternity clothes during five pregnancies. We had a limited clothing budget, and I made many of my clothes myself. I had tried buying cheap clothes but learned to hate them; they fit poorly and were poorly constructed. So, as often as possible, I'd buy more expensive things and fill in with clothes I'd made. I continue to do this, and except for the fact that I sometimes get tired of the same old things, I feel that nice old clothes are nice old friends. How like my mother I've become!

It took me a long time to realize that I did not have to conform to the latest style, and that, in fact, there were some styles and shapes I'd just never do well in but up until the 1960s fashion was quite rigid. Women were still usually doing what they were told, and I really believed I should have had curly hair.

I looked my best and felt the best about my appearance when I was in my mid-30s to late 40s. At that point, my life no longer had to be devoted entirely to my children, and I was beginning to develop a professional life and a persona of my own. I also had more disposable income to spend on my wardrobe, and so I spent more. My outfits were more pulled together, and all those experiments with various "looks" were beginning to pay off. At the same time that I had less need to conform to the latest fashion, fashion in general had become much more permissive.

Once I figured it out, a good-looking suit, pretty blouse or shirt, and comfortable pumps were an easy uniform for business and required little worry. No neckties for me, though. I had been listening to men complain about theirs for so many years and I realized how stupid it would be to fall into the same trap. Otherwise, as long as I wore the colors that were flattering to me, I seemed to always look fine. I wasn't a fashion pacesetter, but I had a pretty and pulled-together look.

The only other event that has affected my looks in the past decade was when I stopped smoking and gained a great deal of weight. After four years, I continue to hope that this is not a permanent condition!

Generally speaking, my friends compliment the clothes I wear when I have taken some time and care with them, and they kindly say nothing when I haven't. I find that it takes a lot of time and care to look the way I'd like to, and I'm not always willing or able to spend that time. I wish looking great were easy and that my closet were full of the right things, all appealing and well-fitting. I wish I looked wonderful all the time without doing any work.

I've seen women who look absolutely smashing—simply dressed but elegant. They make it all look so effortless, but I know that's not true. I've talked with people who have turned the perfection of their appearance into a full-time occupation. One woman told me that in a single week (maybe every week?), she had been to her personal trainer, hairdresser, manicurist, someone for waxing, even an eyebrow person. It worked for her. When she walked into a room, conversation stopped! But that's not for me! There's a nagging, guilty feeling if I devote too much time or money to the process. My parents always emphasized that it was the inner person who counted. As a whole, I think I've devoted far less time and energy to my appearance than to my family and career, and it shows. It's always fun, however, to manage to look really nice, and then see the surprise on people's faces when they find out that I've done some interesting and difficult things in my life.

I'm not sure there's much you can do about the aging process. Certainly plastic surgery is out of the question for me; even the idea terrifies me. I would like to think that as I age, the wrinkles will arrange themselves into pleasing patterns, hopefully reflecting a life well lived, and that I'll have enough money to buy clothes that disguise whatever figure faults develop.

Is there a gap between my mirror image and my self-image? Yes, often. I carry with me some very old-fashioned baggage, maybe as the result of my mother's admonitions. For me, these days, looking like a lady sometimes means looking like an old lady.

B A R B A R A, 65:
fashion illustrator

My first memory of myself was at age 4, when I looked in a tall mirror and said, "I really am an adult now!" I came from a family of all adults and I just felt like one of them. I certainly didn't see myself as a baby, and that was a positive realization.

I was the youngest child, much younger than both my brother, who is seventeen years older than I, and my sister, who is twenty years older. I was lavished with attention and cherished by my parents. I also had very beautiful red hair. The rest of me was a complete disaster, but when people saw me they said, "What gorgeous hair that kid has!" So I grew up thinking that my only asset was my long red hair. All people talked about was my hair, which was very thick, very red, and very long. Nobody ever talked about how bright I was, how pleasant I was, my eyes, my nose, or my legs. So those comments were a negative experience, although no one meant them that way. I cut off my hair as soon as I became a real adult at age 12 because I wanted to look more like other people who weren't redheads!

Otherwise I thought I was brilliant, and because I grew up in a house full of adults, everything I said was repeated and marvelled at. How could this small child say such brilliant things? I didn't even have any peers, because we lived in an area where there were no other kids.

At the same time, however, my mother gave me a very low opinion of myself. She was a very fanciful lady and if I got an A in one subject, she would say, "My daughter got all A's." She had problems in her own life: going through the Great Depression and dealing with a very bad accident that my father had suffered. She received her pleasures by talking about her children, and she would exaggerate my popularity, my talent, my ability in school, and, later, my salary. As a result, I always thought there was something wrong with me. During my teen years and high school, I felt I had to fulfill my parents' expectations, so I chose friends who had some very winning aspects to their lives.

I remember visiting Greenwich Village and the garment district in Manhattan for the first time, and comparing myself with all the fashionable people and wondering, "Why aren't I like them?" So instead of going to college like my sister and brother did, I stuffed my bra and got a job. I wanted to be part of another experience. I was only about 14 or 15 when I met the man I later married at age 17. I was concerned about what was happening at home and this person came into my life, so I simply married him.

I am an illustrator. And no matter what age you are, the art world is competitive. Although I want people to notice me, I also want to disappear "into the woodwork" sometimes. A good way to stay in the woodwork is not to dress, but if you don't dress at all people look at you as unimportant. If you dress as attractively as you can, you are still in the woodwork—just a more attractive piece of it. So I find it's easier to stay in the woodwork looking better than looking worse.

I have pretty much transformed myself in the past few years and people often comment on the results, but I still don't believe them; the compliments embarrass me. It will take a long time for my self-image to catch up with my new exterior. If my artwork gets better, then my self-image may get better, but it still isn't where I want it to be. When it gets there, watch out! I hope.

Anyone who has made as many changes as I have recently needs some time to integrate them all. I need to get used to that new picture of myself in my mind, and I still have a long way to go. When I worked at a large company I thought strictly about the work, not about how to be pleasing visually. I just did my job; I worked hard. But now, as a freelance artist, I want to do what I like, not what *they* like. That's the difference between then and now. It's a big step for me, and these things don't happen overnight. I'm a work in progress.

The best thing that has happened to me is that I no longer care if my knees are knobby or my nose is big. I would like them to be nicer, but I now feel the total look is much more important. It doesn't matter if I am tall or short, fat or thin. I am now more interested in finding the right shoe for the outfit and getting the overall visual line that pleases me. When I do that, I am content, but it is not easy for me. Sometimes I change shoes three times to achieve the total look.

I am much more comfortable with myself now. I used to look at others and try to adopt some of their sense of style, but I don't think that way anymore. It's more important to find my own look and my own comfort level rather than borrow from others. The Japanese designers got me thinking. The Japanese look is so easy; you don't have to think, just move in the clothes.

The most important thing to me now is to look interesting, and I have had some good feedback about myself lately. In the past couple of years I have achieved this appearance goal. Yet, as an artist, I always feel there is a better way to do it with the right sweater, or shoes, or portfolio that I never seem to have. The same thing is true in my work. My wastepaper basket is overflowing; I do the work over and over and over again. It's very hard to please me, but sometimes I do.

When I was married to Mike, the people we knew were different from my friends now. No one ever complimented me when I tried to achieve an interesting or ethnic style. Now people ask me, "Where did you get that scarf? Who's your hairdresser? May I see your portfolio of work?" And they wouldn't ask if they weren't interested. Learning to do all these things on my own has been a big challenge.

I am beginning to learn who I am, what I can do, what I like—not what somebody thinks I should like. Somehow I wasn't able to do that when I was married and working for a big company. My life revolved around what I thought was necessary. But now that I am alone, I have had to stop and think, "What do I want?

I don't know the tricks to selling myself and my work yet, because I never did it before. I am still afraid to say, "Look at this wonderful thing I did." I may think it's wonderful, but it doesn't sound right for me to say it. I have to learn more presentation skills and I think that when I have more confidence in my work, it will be easier for me to market my talent.

I am happier with myself now, but I miss Mike and I am angry that I didn't do this while he was still alive. I let all that time go by just being a "good girl." Not that I should have been bad, but I should have paid more attention to who I was. At times I wish he were here to see me now, but there are other times when I know he wouldn't like some of the "new me." When he would come home from a business trip, he would say, "God, Barbara, you do such beautiful things to our home!" But I would do things only when he was gone, so I guess I was afraid of him and didn't know it.

I am planning on getting my face done in January! The doctor spoke about straightening my nose, which I have to think about. Most of the changes I want to make in my life have to do with my career and accomplishments, but I also hope to stay looking as good as I can and to meet somebody who can be a companion to me. I think a man and a woman need to compromise a lot for a relationship, but as long as they remain individuals, they can compromise for the togetherness. So I hope to meet somebody. But I plan to keep on having fun, joining artists' groups, working, doing my illustrations, and planning my face lift!

Yoji Yamamoto, the Japanese designer, describes himself as "a dressmaker with a little bit of outlaw." I would like to describe myself as a little bit of an outlaw; I feel I need more of that.

B E T H, 47:

junior high mathematics teacher

I am the youngest of four girls, with twin sisters two years older and another sister three and a half years older. As the smallest and youngest child, in this crunch of four girls, I had two hand-me-down dresses to choose from: one was red, the other was blue. I didn't have any new clothes of my own until sixth grade. I didn't think about it positively or negatively; it just was. We were all kind of cute kids and we saw ourselves that way.

I came from a relatively poor family. My parents were the first from their families to have a college education at state teachers' colleges on the East Coast. None of my grandparents went past junior high or spoke grammatical English.

Because we didn't have money, my parents didn't spend on anything. They made do; they bought bargains; they bought things that didn't fit and altered them. I was married before I realized that you could shop until you found clothes that fit—that you could just keep trying things on until you found the right thing.

As a kid, my self-image had to do with how I was perceived by my father, who is very controlling and verbally abusive. I watched what my sisters did and adjusted my behavior to stay out of trouble. I became the all-time 100 percent pleaser; I learned to behave in a way that kept the situation placid. I never said what I felt or asked for what I wanted. I told my parents just enough to keep them from asking more questions. My parents describe me as easygoing, and it's a sick joke. I was Miss Goody Two-shoes. And that's bad. To this day I don't argue with my father. I used to try, and it's not that I want to give in to his point of view, but it's not worth it.

My oldest sister, Kara, who was petite and tiny-boned, was always very picky about clothes. As a college student, she announced she wanted a Lanz dress or nothing for Christmas. Lanz dresses were way out of my parents' price range. But Kara would rather have nothing than something she didn't want. So she got the Lanz dress and we all got things we didn't want.

Kara was a strong person with conservative style. What she said about what I wore had the most influence on me until after I was married. She would make me think subliminally that what she had was what I wanted. All through junior high, high school, and freshman year in college, I wanted her to like what I wore.

At 5'2" with an average bone structure, I could never have emulated my sister Jane, who was 5'7" and had a gorgeous figure. I didn't want to dress like my sister Kayla, who was always in trouble with my parents. She was a little heavy with a bust, and she wore cinched-in waists, crinolines, and spiked heels. She looked pretty bad. She tried eye makeup in high school and got kicked out of the house. That was just not done; "streetwalker" was the name for that look. My mother wasn't an inspiration, either; she was very inconsistent in her taste.

Kara, sweet loving sister, had convinced me that I was fat because she was so thin and small-boned. One time, as a junior in high school, I went swimming with Kara, who commented about a girl who was thinner than I was: "Why would she want to be seen in public in a bathing suit?" Kara had so much influence on me that I believed if she thought that girl was heavy, she must have thought I was heavy too—therefore I must be. The things we do to ourselves and allow others to do to us!

When I got married during senior year in college, my sister Kara made both my wedding dress and her bridesmaid dress. I weighed 115 pounds when I got married, which is certainly not heavyset. But Kara convinced me I should wear a short wedding dress because she was taller than I was and the proportion of my dress would look too wide compared with hers when we were at the altar. So I said "Fine!" How could I have started out in life like that? Today I don't just go along, but it was fine in those days.

Because of Kara, I believed I was "fat" until fifteen years ago. So I grew up with a fat person's mindset, making a typical fat person's comments. In those days, too, I always wore a girdle, which didn't even make sense because I never wore straight slinky skirts that needed a girdle. I now understand that I'm not fat; I've never been fat. I just have a different bone structure than Kara.

I didn't have enough money to dress like other kids in high school; then too, they had totally different figures than I did. I didn't have a real great self-image in high school. Luckily, clothing wasn't as important in those days. I knitted some nice sweaters and I made most of my clothes—A-line skirts with matching round-collared blouses—out of Liberty of London fabric. Although I didn't know how to adjust the patterns well enough to fit me, I could sew quite well; but I had only a few outfits.

For the longest time, I was overly careful about every clothing purchase. I'd shop for something I liked, then find a pattern and make it. I sewed but still wished that I could buy it instead of make it. Luckily I had one really good friend who had a very easygoing attitude about shopping. She bought things and never worried about the money. She taught me that if something looks good on me, I should buy it. During these shopping expeditions, we even got over the hurdle of our different figure types, which were exact opposites.

There were 320 kids in my New Jersey public high school class. I was one of the top students, and the kids I went around with were bright just like me. I didn't dare go around with any other crowd. My parents would say very disparaging things about other kids: "Isn't it dreadful, so-and-so teases her hair and she's going out for cheerleading!" If the girl under discussion was someone I was friendly with, my parents' opinion nixed the friendship real quick.

Someone once asked me if I had been a cheerleader. Well, I was in the Honor Society, and Honor Society members did not go out for cheerleading! Not in my family! It wasn't allowed, even though I had the personality. My father said the word "cheerleader" in the same tone of voice that he said "stewardess" and "nurse"! Dancers were not even talked about—they were totally unacceptable. I was literally brainwashed into believing that appearance, intellect, and personality couldn't all be part of the same package. If you spent time or money on clothes, you were decadent.

With all that, I think my self-image started to change when I was about 30 years old. I finally decided that I wasn't like my family and that was okay. However, I still wasn't the person I am now. I was still a goody-goody who was competent at what I did, and who didn't swear in public or make waves of any kind.

I definitely feel I dress better than ever at the present. Now I buy clothes that fit. I don't love to shop, but I like fun things to wear and I no longer care what my family thinks about the expense. My parents would faint if they knew what I spend on clothes or how much enjoyment I get out of them. After all these years, those two controlling people still say things like, "She spends an awful lot of money on clothes!" in a tone of voice that implies mortal sin. They have all kinds of reasons why I shouldn't spend my hard-earned money.

Now I wear what I want when I'm with my parents. Before I turned thirty, I would have either dressed down or lied about the price, but I don't care anymore. If they think we're spendthrifts, or my children have too much, or that we make too much money, I can't help it. Mother says in her best manner, "Well, you're certainly out of my league!" What can I say to that? They spend their money the way they want, but they don't acknowledge other people's right to do the same.

So spending money on appearance *per se* was viewed very negatively in our family. And as far as my parents are concerned, it still is. They just don't do that kind of thing. I've had to get through a lot in order to enjoy life and its treats.

One of the problems I've had to overcome is the idea that intelligent, academic people can also spend money on clothes and good looks. My family's viewpoint was that academics—where you went to school, and how well you did—were THE most important things. My sisters and I were ranked according to our academic performance; and any of our classmates who didn't rank in the top 10 percent were lumped into the group that "spent a lot of time on their appearance or were cheerleaders!" I can't even duplicate the tone of voice my parents used on that sentence.

It's amazing how parental attitudes get beaten into you and stay with you for so long. Because my parents didn't consider it important for intelligent people to be well-dressed, if anyone complimented me on my clothing I felt it was a negative. I didn't want to be taken for an airhead! Why appearance and intellect couldn't go together, I'm not quite sure. But I've gotten over that.

I finally broke out of the rut. I started finding clothes I liked. Then I realized there was "fun stuff" out there that I could have. I started getting compliments on things which my conservative friends claim I would never have worn before! So in getting rid of all the other boundaries, I have gotten rid of the need to wear only tailored, professional clothes. I still don't wear diaphanous skirts, because you know what "kind of people" wear those! But I am having more fun finding all kinds of artsy things.

It was never like that growing up. One did not have fun dressing oneself. The last thing I want to do now is look like anybody else. In high school I very much wanted to look like my perception of everybody else but I couldn't even do that; we couldn't afford it. When I started to buy things on my own, I wanted to be safe and look intelligent. Nothing sexy, nothing alluring, that was not done. Even now, it's not my personality, but if I happen to see something I like that might be alluring, I won't necessarily pass it up. I'll find an occasion to wear it with my husband.

These days, I am a much more relaxed, even frivolous person, and it doesn't fight with my intellect. I try a lot more things. It's my turn to be captain of the tennis team this summer. I want to get out on Rollerblades!

With the kids gone, I am much more relaxed; I can entertain and not have to cook all the food. I can buy stuff. Who cares? I don't feel I have to prove anything or apologize for anything. It is thrilling to give up some of this mythology. Those are the changes I want to keep working on in my life. I am less time-oriented and devote more time to myself. Being busy all the time with work and social life doesn't do it for me; I don't need the social roller-coaster.

I personally think that I look better than ever. There's a wonderful Doonesbury cartoon in which Joanie is waiting for "the call" from Clinton, hoping she will be part of the cabinet. Frame after frame, she is waiting for the call. And in the last frame she says, "This is just like junior high, but now I have my hair figured out!" To me that says it all. I've got my clothes figured out, my hair is low-maintenance now, and I've had my teeth capped. And because I feel I've gotten better-looking, I don't think I'm threatened by the aging process. So far. I don't want to gain any weight. I've gotten rid of my fat person's mentality. That's what I'm doing with myself. Tah Dah!!!

C A R O L, 49 :

corporate manager

I remember myself, mostly through the family pictures, as a child with blonde curly hair. I always liked my first-grade picture because my hair was long. Normally I don't photograph well; I just freeze in front of a camera, probably because I'm so self-conscious about being photographed. Other than that I have a fairly good self-image.

My first memories of myself are of a very independent, self-reliant, and assertive child. When I was 4 years old, we lived a couple of blocks from the downtown area, and when I wanted to go downtown I just went. The neighbors often retrieved me, asking, "What are you doing downtown?"

I would have hated to be my mother and to have to put up with my antics. I remember being in a movie theater once with my older sister and some neighbor kids. I didn't like the movie so I got up and walked out. When the usher said, "Where are you going?" I said, "I'm going home. I don't like the movie!" When he told me I couldn't go home, I said, "Yes, I can!" And I went. I did stuff like that constantly.

When I was in kindergarten, we moved to a different neighborhood with the grammar school some distance from where we lived. My mother took me to school the first day and said she would come and get me when class let out. I said, "That won't be necessary." She said, "Well, you'll have to take the bus home." I said, "I can do that. You don't have to come and get me." Mother finally said, "All right!" So I went home on the bus by myself from my first day in kindergarten. That's how my childhood went because I have always preferred doing things myself rather than having other people do them for me.

I have succeeded in most of the things I have done; I don't remember doing anything that didn't work or anything that absolutely flopped. So I don't really remember any negative feelings about growing up. One of the nuns in grade school always told us, "Don't go through life without trying everything. Don't say you can't do it. Give it a try!" I have lived by that motto. As a result, I have never had problems meeting people, tackling new projects or jobs, going off on my own, or travelling by myself.

Occasionally in grade school or high school I wasn't in the right group. I do remember it being very difficult to change schools when I was in fifth grade. I was queasy about venturing into that new setting; but it wasn't so much fear as apprehension about whether the kids would like me. We always want to be liked at that age. Well, we still do!

I never thought I was cute, but once in grade school my friend Pat said, "Do you know who my brother thinks is the cutest girl in our class?" I had always idolized Pat's older brother, John; everyone thought he was just a dream. So I named a bunch of the cute girls. And then Pat said, "You!" I said, "Me?" I thought I looked all right, but I never perceived myself as being the best-looking in the class.

I enjoyed myself in high school and had a very good self-image. I always played a leadership role in the student council and the high school musicals. I did not like to perform, however; I always stayed in the background running the stage crew and doing all that behind-the-scenes work. That took a lot of energy. I also worked a part-time job all through high school. Initially I did baby-sitting and light housework for a family; later I clerked at our neighborhood hardware store.

In high school I dated a fellow named Wayne who was a very poor choice on my part, although I didn't realize it. None of my friends liked him, but they didn't say much to me. Although the school guidance counselor tried to clue me in with prompts from my girlfriends, it wasn't until I started college that I understood Wayne didn't fit in the picture. We quickly went our separate ways and I was able to avoid making a big mistake.

During my college years, I perceived myself as being very ambitious. When I met with my adviser for the first time, I told him I intended to go through school in three years and he said, "There is no way!" So I said, "You watch me!" I programmed my curriculum myself because I was going to get through in three years if it killed me. Talk about a challenge. His comment assured me that I would accomplish my plan. It wasn't a difficult school and elementary education was not a hard major. I went directly into my college courses that first summer out of high school and also attended classes the following two summers. I continued to work part-time at the hardware store, too. I didn't find it difficult; it was just enough of a challenge. After college, marriage, and return to the work force, I earned master's degrees in Library Science and Business Administration. People always comment on why I keep getting more degrees. It's the challenge; I like to keep busy and keep my mind active.

I got married a couple of years out of college, but if I had it to do over again I'd never get married that young. I keep telling my kids to find out who they are first and discover their interests. They will develop differently if they allow themselves that time. In college you and your spouse-to-be may feel you're compatible and interested in the same things just because you're both in college, but as years go by that does not necessarily continue.

I don't know why, but I have always felt more comfortable with men than women. Maybe my working in the hardware store brought that out. I have found through the years that I am closer friends with men than women. I am very competitive, too. One of the things about teaching that I didn't care for was the mostly-women environment. The same was true with library work, which I did for a while after getting my master's degree in library science. Even when I worked at the local university extension as non-library staff, there were enough women there that I couldn't relate to the atmosphere. I wanted to be in a more businesslike setting. Finally, when I moved to a job as librarian at an engineering firm that was almost all men, I felt very comfortable.

I used to have a mole on the side of my nose, which I did not have removed until I was almost 40 years old. When I went to the dermatologist and asked him to take it off, he said, "You must have a very good self-image to have lived with a mole in that spot all these years! Why are you coming in now? Why didn't you come in when you were 20?" I did it only because everyone was bugging me that it might become cancerous. Before that I never gave it a thought. If it hadn't been for the cancer scare, I would probably still have the darn mole.

I have always perceived myself as being somewhat overweight, and have dreamed of being 10 to 20 pounds lighter. The only time I was ever at my ideal weight was when I worked for the park system during the summers in college. After I was married, I went to T.O.P.S., took off a few pounds, and was quite slender for a while. Of course, I got sick, so that ended that. I have always thought that I should be slimmer, so my only real image problem has been my weight.

I've always had a lot of self-confidence and I still do. I never cared for the fact that I was always a few pounds overweight, but I guess I also have a phobia about aging. Fortunately I come from a family that doesn't have a tendency to go gray or to wrinkle. Of course, with fat cheeks and a little flesh on, you don't show the wrinkles so much.

Exercise is something I should get into, but I haven't motivated myself enough to do it. I think people who stay physically fit and trim really look good. If I lost a few pounds and got into shape, I would feel better about my appearance and perhaps wear better clothes. But that has not affected my self-confidence at work or in general.

I am definitely comfortable with myself—with where I am, what I'm doing, and how I am getting along in the world. I am very outgoing which helps in the business world as well as personally. I also have a very good rapport with people. I have never run into anyone I couldn't work with; I have always found a way to get along with co-workers. Every now and then there might be a real pistol out there who made other people say they couldn't work with him or her. I try to be a little more tactful or approach each person a little differently. And that's always been a real asset in any job, as far as I'm concerned.

I think others perceive me as a leader and expect a lot of me. I was very encouraged at my current corporate position when I was offered the opportunity to change career paths. The company is investing a lot of money in training me. My employers had the confidence that I'd quickly pick up my new responsibilities.

I am basically happy with the person I am today. If I had it to do over again, I would start developing my business skills a lot earlier; I would not stay home with my children as long as I did. I like to see mothers stay home with their kids when they're little, but I also think that career women need to balance things. Young mothers give up a lot these days if they hold off on careers for which they've been educated. It's a very competitive world out there. I could have gone a lot farther in the corporate world than I will ultimately be able to go if I had started earlier. I am competing with people who have twenty-five years experience, when I have only six, and I just can't make up for all those years. Plus, I think my kids would have been more independent had I gone back to work and put more responsibility on them earlier. But I guess I have to look at where my generation is coming from. Neither my mother nor my husband's mother ever worked.

I didn't go to college with the idea that I was going have a career. I just went. I took an education degree—one of the degrees that girls usually took in those days. I got married. I didn't plan far enough ahead. And if you don't use your career skills, they are going to be lost by the time you go back to work. You can't have a ten- or fifteen-year gap in your work experience and then jump right back in and say, "Here I am again." You have to start over and build from a new foundation.

I didn't work when my kids were very little. Once they both got into grade school, I became a substitute teacher, which convinced me that teaching was definitely not for me. I absolutely had to do something different. At that point, I had gotten into genealogy as an avocation and had a lot of exposure to libraries. Library science was the only master's degree

I could get without a lot of prerequisites and extensive commuting because many of those classes were offered here in town. In addition, I still had the kids at home and all kinds of family obligations. Thinking that I could fit in and enjoy working in the library world, I took the master's degree. But if I had it to do all over again, I would do that differently also. It was not a good move on my part. Had I researched the program better and known more about it, I would never have done what I did.

I still have enormous family obligations all the time. And now since my dad has died, I feel that I am obligated to look out for my mother and be with her more. Not that she's not capable, but I go over to see her every other night and call on the telephone more often. It takes a lot of extra time. And then there's all the other obligations at home: cooking family dinners and entertaining relatives. I feel I have to have my mother and mother-in-law over every so often. I have so many "have-to's." Someday, I'd like to pick up and just say, "Hey, I'm off!" And away I'd go to do my own thing.

But this is all part of how I was raised. My mother always had my grand-mother over for dinner every week as a regular event. And on holidays my mother always entertained family. I have all these built-in obligations that I was raised with and it's hard to break out of the mold. It's hard to say, "Hey, deep down I don't really want to do all this stuff." But I can't just walk out on it. Well, I could walk out on it but then I'd have to live with the guilt. But I can fantasize!

The other day I was going through some old photographs when I found one of me as May Queen in grade school. The May Queen was chosen by election and I won by one vote—because I voted for myself. Our teacher had given us a lecture on voting procedures. "When you run for election, if you feel you are qualified, you should vote for yourself. If you don't think you're qualified, who will?" So I voted for myself. I beat out a girl named Mary by one vote; I have always felt kind of guilty about that!

POSTSCRIPT: After thirty years of marriage, Carol did walk out of her demanding situation, was married again to a very compatible partner, retired from a major corporation at age 54 and is now spending winters in Florida, summers in Wisconsin. She works part-time at whatever job is appealing and flexible. Life is great!

CARON, 50:

community volunteer

My first memory of my appearance is of my maternal grandfather's negative criticism. He told me I had bowlegs. I was shocked when he said that; it's not as if I went out and got bowlegs on purpose. But he also said I looked good in a particular outfit, and that was positive. So I learned that people are critical of you. My grandfather pointed out my negatives and also my positives. Those incidents happened during my awkward stage, when I was not particularly cute. You'd think that my family would have been more helpful, but they weren't.

That grandfather was the patriarch of the family, and if he said something, wasn't it true? My mother was always very critical, too. Learning that my appearance could be criticized made me self-conscious, a trait I have carried throughout my life. I learned there could be something "wrong" with my appearance. There was a right way to look, a wrong way to look; a right thing to do, a wrong thing to do. I became uncomfortable with any praise. I was almost more comfortable with the criticism because I could fight back; the praise was hard to accept. I recently read that most people are more comfortable with their own negative thinking than with positive thinking. So we all tend to fall into that pattern. But why can't we feel good about ourselves? "Self-praise stinks!" is a German phrase my mother always used.

During early childhood and adolescence, I was very athletic. That gave me a positive sense of self because I felt very safe in athletics. But my mother was not athletic and considered it something one "didn't do." I was a good swimmer and really liked swimming, but Mother said to stop because I was developing broad shoulders and would soon look like a milkmaid! I realize, now, of course, that people don't get broad shoulders from swimming but through heredity. Mine came from my father.

I never really knew what being female meant and I felt very inhibited. Mother never gave me a clear picture of what it meant to be female. I only knew that you didn't want to be too "suggestive." God only knows what that was, but I didn't want to be that. I knew what I shouldn't do but not what I should do. That was from my mother's point of view, and she was the dominant person in our family. She decided what we could do and what we couldn't do. She did the best she could, I suppose, but she could never see any other way. She could never listen, or believe there was another side to any story. My father encouraged me, but only as much as men encouraged girls to do anything in those days. Unfortunately, my father didn't have much effect on my self-esteem.

I saw myself as different, which only made me more tentative. I had already realized that the rules in my house were different from the rules in other kids' houses. For example, I went to other kids' houses and played in their bedrooms, but I couldn't have kids over to visit, and they couldn't come into my bedroom to play. When I asked my mother why, she said, "Nice people don't have other people in to play in their bedrooms!" I also never slept over at anybody's house; we "just didn't do that."

I have no sensitivities to my physical characteristics—none at all! I have a nose I hate, a chin that's no good, and I'd like to have had braces on my teeth. I wish I had a better hairline and healthier nails. I feel okay about my legs, though, after all these years. And there's nothing I'm going to rush out and have done unless they lower the price of all these repair jobs.

I never had sensitivities in grade school because I was so physically active. Then, too, I was thin; my sister was fat. It was "not good" to be fat; my grandfather had said so. By being heavy, my sister saved me a lot of grief. She took a lot of the heat. Thank God my sister was fat, because my only positive stroke was that I wasn't fat!

During early teenage years and high school, I was very sheltered. My mother's rules kept me away from the other kids pretty effectively. I could see some of my old grade school classmates becoming very popular, and it was clear to me that I was not one of the popular kids. As a result, I was very intimidated, very unsure of how to act with them. I had a few good girlfriends, but I wasn't in the big group of popular kids that hung around together.

I always had boyfriends and dates. Dating and popularity with boys was not a big issue for me in high school. Boys were okay for me. I grew up and played with boys my whole life because we didn't live near any girls my age. My mother didn't want to hear about boys, though. And if I had some ideas about boys, she'd dismiss them, saying, "What dime novels are you reading now?"

I worried more about fitting in with the girls. I didn't quite know how to relate to girls and that caused me much anxiety. I never felt that I could make the transition from dealing with boys to dealing with girls.

It is interesting that my mother felt very uncomfortable with women herself, but she would never admit it. I didn't learn one thing from her about getting along with other women. My sense of myself with other women is less positive than with men. I am much more comfortable, more at ease, with men.

All these family issues fed into my sense of appearance, which was very tentative on some levels. To this day, put me in sports clothes, please! I know sports clothes and I feel comfortable in them. But out there in the more dressed-up, "grown-up" women's world, I am terribly unsure of myself. I don't know what looks good on me; I don't have a feel for that. But sports clothes, yes. That's what worked for me as a kid. And I stuck with sports clothes because they worked for me.

When I went away to college, I went wild because I had no framework of behavior. Absolutely nothing. And I couldn't talk to my mother because I didn't think she knew either. She never said, "I don't know; maybe we can talk about it." If she didn't know, it wasn't important. She was very dismissive and very defensive. My mother was not a role model for successful social interaction—she was a role model for a recluse!

In college, I had terrific roommates who really helped me. They were not really popular, either, but they felt the same way I did, and at last we could talk about it. I really lucked out with these good friends. I was never in a sorority, because I never felt comfortable enough to go through Rush. That fear of being rejected was so overwhelming that I couldn't do it, but my roommates were never in a sorority either. Years later, when my daughter went through Rush, I thought how brave she was, but I did not tell her that the whole idea of Rush had been very hard for me.

David, my husband, whom I met in college, was really helpful to me, too. He focused me. I had gotten okay grades in high school without trying, but my first year in college, I went wild and didn't study. When I started dating David, we studied together. And the resulting good grades helped my self-image, because then I was smart. But my mother and father were never impressed with my accomplishments in college. I don't really know what they expected, to tell you the truth!

For me, the most important factor in going away to college was getting away from my mother's influence. That was the good part. The bad part was when I graduated and wanted to get an apartment away from home; it was absolutely not allowed. My mother said, "No, don't do that. That is stupid. Save your money!" I didn't know why I needed to save money, though. I couldn't spend it on anything. I wasn't allowed to buy a car; I wasn't allowed to live away from home because "nice girls don't do that."

Going back home after I graduated from college was the worst experience of my life. I went to work, came home, went to my room, and stayed there. I spent the whole first year in my room. I talked to no one. I became so isolated that I was terrified to meet people I didn't know, even David's graduate school friends. And this was after I had been away at college for four years! At this point in my life, I would have to say I've made some positive steps in spite of the fact that I never felt unconditional acceptance in my family—I felt approved of in some areas, but not all. If I hadn't married David, I'd still be there in my room. No, I'd be with Mom in the nursing home—in the bed next to her!

My self-image is much more positive now, because I have come to grips with who I am and with who I am never going to be. And that's okay. More important, I've come to grips with who my mother is. She is someone who is never going to change, and that's okay now, too. So, I have made changes that make me feel more comfortable about myself. I have now taken control of some situations that were truly awful.

The biggest thing in my life was coming to grips with my mother and all her rules, and realizing that, although they are true for her, they are not true for me. Bringing those feelings to the forefront has been a long and arduous process; but now I can decide what I want, not what I'm "supposed to do." And I can believe that I deserve it. That does a lot for my self-image.

I had to make these changes in myself because my life was just so uncomfortable! But how I did it, beats me. Going to graduate school got me out of the house after David and I got married. Majoring in psychology was no happenstance—I was really working on myself. That helped a lot. And then having kids forced me to get out. I had no choice but to meet other women and mothers. And that gave me a little practice and some insight into how other women do things.

Fortunately my feelings about women have also changed. As I grew older, I learned to deal with women successfully on a one-to-one basis, and now I have some very good friendships with women. But social events with crowds of women still terrify me. I feel I don't have the right thing on; I don't know what to say; I don't know how to make chitchat comfortably. But if I take women individually or in small groups, I am fine. So my self-image is getting better in that respect, even if I'm still unsure of myself at times.

In my late 30s, I came to the conclusion that my nose will never be small and cute, my poor chin will always be the same, and my teeth, unless I do something about them, will never be lined up nicely. That's how it is and I guess I feel okay. I would describe myself as a wholesome, comfortable person. And now I can even dress up! I can do that now, when I want to. Mostly I am comfortable—even though my legs will never be any longer. Isn't it awful? You look at Cindy Crawford in all those magazines and then you have to look at yourself in the mirror every day.

I think I feel better than ever about the way I look, although my kids have pointed me out in old pictures as an absolute geek. When you're a kid your parents say you're ugly, and when you're older your kids say you're ugly! But I definitely think I look better now. I know I'm getting older and it shows, but I feel better than ever, because I like myself better. God, I'm just twenty-five years too late!

I feel fairly integrated in appearance, intellect, and personality. It's all working out. I would still like to be taller, and fix some things about myself, so there is a gap between the mirror image and my self-image. But in my heart of hearts I really feel okay these days. Besides, I don't know what I'd do if I woke up tall and gorgeous! Nobody would recognize me!

When I'm having a good hair day, it would be great if someone said, "Caron, your hair looks great!" And if I look good, I wish someone would say so. But now I am able to ask for reinforcement. I can say to David and the kids, "Don't I look good?" And they have no choice but to say yes. I think people you see every day just don't see you anymore. You are just there, so they don't bother with compliments. I wish my family would notice me more, not take me so for granted.

How do others see me? I think they see me as open, and comfortable, and intellectually probing. And honest. I try to be as honest as possible because I value honesty in others. However, I'm not really sure I know how other people perceive me; most people don't say. And I am so defensive that I can't read others on that issue.

I am happy with who I am today. Any big changes? I feel that changes will just happen and they'll work out. I will deal with the aging process one day at a time. Sometimes I wonder if I should feel older than I do, especially on those days when I get up feeling great, energetic, and young. And then I look in the mirror and see these little lines and this sagging face. I look 50, but I feel younger than my chronological age. Fifty sounds old; 50 used to be one foot in the grave. I don't feel old. Maybe we don't have to be old at 50; there's no reason to be. However everybody around me who is 50 looks 45!

If I could change one thing about myself, I'd like to be slower-paced. I have always operated in fits and starts, racing to get things done, and I don't want to be so reactive anymore. I want to calm down and be my own person. Here I am again, twenty-five years too late. Will I ever get it?

CHRIS, 36:
full-time wife and mother

My parents called me Pixie because I was small with really short hair. I was a real peanut, but because I thought I was cute, I didn't mind being called Pixie. All I ever wanted was long hair like the other girls, but my mother always had my hair cut really short. Every time we went to get my hair cut, I felt butchered but when I finally let my hair grow long, it was unattractive on me. So the first sense I had of myself not looking so good was with longer hair which just didn't do what it was supposed to do. I was better off with that short pixie haircut. Maybe I should have thanked my mother all those years!

I have no recollection of my parents or relatives giving me any sense of positive self-image. And even though I was really little, I didn't have any sensitivities toward physical traits or personality traits until I realized that nobody wanted a puny, unathletic kid on their team. So childhood incidents that contributed to my sense of identity were not so much about how I looked but about sports and friends. The more I wasn't picked for teams and the more I wasn't chosen as someone's best friend, the more my self-image suffered.

Not only did my parents not encourage me to do athletic things, but they also actively discouraged me from doing dangerous or hurtful things. I was, and still am, an incredible swimmer, but that never came into play with other kids. It was the team sports that flummoxed me. I just wasn't a team player then and I'm not one now. That's okay with me at this point, but back then nobody ever said it was okay to not play team sports. If you didn't there was only one conclusion—you were less of a person!

By my early teen years, I had gone from being a peanut to being very tall and very thin. When we had our eighth-grade yearbook picture taken, one of the teachers got the idea for a police line-up photo. So he had lines put on the wall for 6', 5'11", 5'10", and so on. There I was in the line-up, as tall and thin as some of the guys and wearing braces. It was devastating!

I felt too that I did not stack up to the other girls because they all matured much earlier than I did. I was almost a year younger than the rest of my class. Everybody else had their periods and breasts and bras; I had no period and no breasts and an undershirt. Unfortunately, I went to elementary school with girls who were all huge-breasted, and it took me a while to come to grips with the fact that those girls had something I didn't have.

Although I never developed huge breasts, I never got negative messages from my father, thank heavens, so that was okay. The father of a friend of mine used to leave *Playboy* magazines all over the house and she still hasn't gotten over her lack of melon-sized breasts. I don't think I have great breasts, but I wouldn't really want them to be pendulous. I enjoy the way I am, but that doesn't negate the fact that women with big breasts get more attention. All the big-breasted girls in my elementary school had all the dates. And yet I feel sorry for girls who get that kind of attention at such a young age.

Finally, on my thirteenth birthday I got my period. And then once I matured and left for boarding school, things were better. Boarding school was the best thing that ever happened to me: I started wearing makeup, shaving my legs, and doing all the things my parents wouldn't let me do. My hair grew out and by the time I hit the eleventh grade I was pretty happy with my looks. I had long brown hair, breasts (albeit small), and a waist. I seemed to be attractive to the guys, although there were only 12 girls to 320 guys, so we couldn't tell if we were really cute or simply female. Because we were allowed to date at school, I ended up dating a lot of guys. It was a good experience; I came away with a pretty good self-image.

I remember that somewhere between Mercersburg Prep School and Vassar I didn't dress with a real sense of myself. I had very nice, very traditional clothes but I didn't wear anything sexy. My clothes were prudish, let's put it that way. While shopping for my graduation formal, a creamy white gown, I was told by the male shopowner that I looked like a vanilla ice cream cone; I thought my mother was going to drop off the chair. That was my first indication that I was anything like sexy.

During my freshman year in college I decided to buy more feminine clothes and to get away from all my unisex corduroys, sweaters, and turtlenecks. Although by then I had a better sense of my own body, I desperately wanted to look like Cheryl Tiegs. I still do! If I could look like anyone, I would change to Cheryl Tiegs in a second. Even though I am confident in my appearance, she was the standard of beauty when I grew up.

I guess a lot of guys thought I was pretty sexy. And a friend's mother once told me that I had "S.A., if you know what that is!" So slowly but surely I was getting a sense that I was a sexual being, which was a real shock since my parents weren't sexual beings at all. Sex was never discussed at home and I'd never considered myself sexy, so it took me aback at first. Getting feedback about how people perceived me and integrating it into my feelings about myself was a real important issue. Most of us don't get enough feedback as to how we are perceived, and many people don't think about it enough to give valid feedback to others.

Apparently, a lot of women feel threatened by me, although I don't think I am a particularly threatening person. Many people have told me that I seem unapproachable—a real snot, a real bitch—until they get to know me. Then they are pleasantly surprised to find that I am very approachable and warm. In reality, I am a snob, so I guess they recognize it. But I am also shy, so I see myself as approachable. Maybe the fact that I'm judgmental is what people sense; I am very hard on people and they know that I am judging them!

I am happy with the way I look. I haven't reached the point where I look in the mirror and think I'm going downhill yet; I think I am still improving. I thought I looked really good when I was younger, but my frame of reference has changed and I have changed my self-image and the way I dress. My mother raised me traditionally and for a long time I dressed that way, nicely but without a sense of style. As a single careerwoman, I dressed very well within the banking industry parameters. When I married and quit working, there were no holds barred and now I tend to wear anything within reason.

Staying abreast of the current styles helps me to feel good about myself. Too many women who feel they look good in college stay with that look until age 40 or more, and then wonder why they have lost their pizzazz when they should have updated all along. When I am creative enough to update my look, then I feel good. I always tell my husband, Rick, that he doesn't have to take a lover because I look different every six months: brownette, then redhead, then blonde! I recently told my hairdresser to cut my hair off-kilter so I won't look like every other mother in the area. I don't want to look like a mother! I am one, to the nth degree, but I am determined not to look as if I have four kids. So many women give in to the mother formula: gain 20 pounds, wear jeans and T-shirts, pull their hair back, and give up on makeup. Others fight it every inch of the way, which is what I am doing. My rebellion has more to do with how I dress than anything. I don't want people to think, "She had four kids and she let herself go!"

I still go in and out of insecure phases about my looks—I'm sure everyone does—but I would describe myself as confident. I think I appear in control and happy with myself. I am aware of who I am, who I want to be, and what suits me. I cringe at the word cute; it's not something I aspire to. I feel I am pleasing-looking but I've always wanted to be drop-dead gorgeous. I don't know if all women want that or not. I'll never get over not looking like Cheryl Tiegs, my icon. These days you see all kinds of beauty in magazines and the models are no longer so thin. It's not so prescribed. I think it's much healthier now than it was when I was growing up.

I look as good as ever these days, although I see myself as a little overweight. I looked better when I worked full-time and taught aerobic dance. I was in incredible shape; that's when I looked my best. But then again, although I liked my body shape, I didn't necessarily like my hair and I wasn't as comfortable with myself as I am now.

My sense of comfort with myself as a whole spills over into an acceptance of myself at this point in life, and it's overridden everything except those several pounds! It's overridden my graying hair (which I camouflage) and the changes in my skin tone. I'm sure it relates to my not wanting to look as if I have had four kids. I don't want people to say, "Oh, you look good for having four kids!," because I will immediately internalize it.

Last year Rick said I was over the line weightwise. This year he said I look really good but just need to get in shape. I guess I am more accepting of myself now, which is why I don't exercise! Exercise becomes stressful because I don't have the time. It's on my list of goals to attain.

Since I've had kids I've had a lot of trouble with my self-image because I don't really have an identity. Very few of the men I know give any weight to homemaking and motherhood. They see working women as more intelligent because they get paid. When I worked I was reviewed every six months and was told I did a great job. I derived a lot of confidence from all that and it's been a long time since I have gotten that kind of qualitative feedback. Although I am confident that I am smart, it's been only in the past few years that I feel more strongly that what I do as a mother is important.

There is a gap between my mirror image and my self-image. Sometimes I think I am a lot more attractive than my mirror image! I always hated my nose, thinking it was too big for my face, but now I've decided I like my nose on my face. I always used to pooh-pooh Rick if he complimented me, thinking, "How could he say that?" But I dismissed his compliments for so long they started coming less often. Now I am gracious when I get a compliment. And Rick reminds me that he wouldn't have married me if I weren't attractive, so if I feel particularly ugly I remind myself of that statement.

These days I'm comfortable enough to not worry if I don't look great; that's a big thing for me. I used to have to be dressed perfectly and made up all the time. However, once you get an integrated picture of yourself, being dressed up or made up isn't quite as important. I am more comfortable in my skin than ever before.

I will need some new "shtick" sooner or later because I feel more important with a salaried job. It's still difficult for me to feel that being home with four kids is totally valid. Intellectually I know it's important and I wouldn't have done it any other way, but I still feel I haven't been validated. A lot of it is our culture, but I know I will have to go back to work to get an identity. Part of me would be happy being June Cleaver, but the message I got at Vassar was, "You are nothing unless you are something." There was certainly no importance given to raising a family, and you couldn't just be something, you had to be INTERESTING! That programming is hard to overcome.

I do like my life, and my four girls are really an important part of it, but I need a new career that's flexible. I could be an important role model for the girls, if I went back to work, even part-time; they would see that mothers are not just people who stay around the house all the time. They might also see that life is divided into segments. You move to a new segment, start experimenting, and take on new things. I want them to see that people don't stay the same. They were excited and very supportive recently when I did a hand modeling job for a photo shoot. So I think it would be very good for them to experience their mother working, especially in something unconventional. And to see the paycheck, too!

The prospect of hand modeling could be fun and the rejection factor is low. Hands are a commodity and they either fit the advertiser 's needs or not. If somebody likes my hands, it's a real kick; if they don't, it's not the end of the world. I couldn't deal with the rejection of my face or body. I consider myself a strong person but I'm too vulnerable when it comes to my body and how others perceive it.

I find that women seldom reinforce each other about their appearance. One of my friends says positive things, but no one else ever tells me that I look great or good or pretty. A guy will, sometimes, although I am not around too many men. A woman's attitude seems to be that if they tell another woman she looks good it makes them less good-looking or it makes the pool of available compliments smaller. However, I recognize the feeling because if Rick says some other woman is intelligent, I often feel that I am therefore less intelligent. Is that just a women's thing? I do, however, go out of my way to tell someone if she looks attractive or if I like her outfit. In the past five years I've become aware that people don't compliment me much, and it makes me wonder why people can comment on clothing but not on a really personal level. The scant compliments from men I can understand; their wives wouldn't allow it! But I don't understand why many women are so unsupportive of each other.

I had no problem turning 30 and I don't see 40 as a problem. Even the thought of 50 doesn't bother me. I think that I will still be attractive and vital. Some women think 30 is time for a face-lift and 40 is the end of the world. Even 60 doesn't frighten me, I don't think, but 70 is getting up there! Maybe in another ten years 70 won't seem so scary. My mother keeps saying that we become ready for each change as it comes along. I plan to be a very striking older woman, attractive and comfortable with myself, whom people look at and say, "Wow, she's terrific!" And maybe that's my problem in finding the words to describe myself now. I am waiting to be a really striking older woman!

Even though I said I would like to look like Cheryl Tiegs, I do think I have gotten it together. I would like to get in shape, but I don't plan on any tummy tucks, face-lifts, or eye lifts unless my eyelids come down over my eyes. If I have gotten over my nose, I can do okay with the other stuff. There's a real beauty in a woman who has grown comfortably into her age, as opposed to fighting it and looking inappropriate. I hope that as I get to a certain age my appearance will become much less important than who I am.

I will be curious to see how my four girls do with their self-esteem, as they are not around boys in school. Maybe they won't get those societal messages pounded into them all the time, although the time will come when they want that feedback from boys, too. It's important. They may be pretty and even know they are pretty, but they will need males to tell them the same thing. There's a lot to be said for not needing that sort of affirmation, which would be the best situation, but I don't know where you get it if you aren't a conventional beauty. My girls seem to be more conventionally pretty than I was; none of them seem to have the gawkiness that I had. I wonder if they will have an easier time because of that.

I see the cultural messages about body image taking hold in my girls, however, from the stupid TV shows. Even the indirect messages are frightening. I purposely have never brought any magazines into the house because magazines are so ridiculous. So maybe having a mother who's confident will make a difference because kids pick that stuff up and identify with it. My mother was a giver; she did everything for everyone else. She was very conventional but frighteningly insecure. She has the worst self-image of anyone I've ever met.

Growing up was horrible for me. I had a very hard time, and most of the women who have discussed this issue with me say the same thing. But curiously, the strongest women I know are the ones who had a difficult experience growing up. I gravitate toward people who are very strong in their own way and who have a very strong sense of who they are. Maybe it's a rite of passage.

COLLEEN, 48:
art consultant, watercolorist

My first memory of myself is from a photograph that floated around the house for years. I hated that picture. I looked urchin-like, with bangs that needed cutting, and my darling little baby sister was in the background. I looked unsure of myself and unhappy with my appearance. In earlier pictures I was a cute little thing, but this one showed my feelings as a young girl growing up with a prettier sibling.

Throughout my childhood, everyone said I looked like my father. That bothered me because I didn't understand that they meant I also had my father's personality and very likable manner. I always saw it as "who wants to look like a man?" Who wants to have this nose? The space between the teeth? And people always commented on my sister, "Oh, isn't Susie cute, she looks just like her mother. And Colleen looks like her dad!" This is something I have dealt with my whole life.

But the positive part was that this neat man, my father, was my closest ally. In my heart, that made up for the fact that I looked "like a man," and I just grew to understand that it wasn't so bad. I am really happy now to have my dad's looks and personality and character. I have the features but also the soul of my father. I treasure that.

I also recall feeling very strongly about my freckles: I hated them! But as I got older, I either got used to the freckles or they faded to the point they didn't bother me anymore. It's amazing what age does. Now I have liver spots and I'd trade them for a few freckles.

As a youngster, I thought my nose seemed too big for my face and it wasn't until much later that I really grew into my nose. I used to pick on my sister and tell her that her gums showed when she smiled. I was always looking for faults in her so that mine wouldn't seem so bad!

I didn't have a figure to speak of. In seventh grade I got a bra because I got all A's on my report card. It had nothing to do with my figure; it was a training bra. Like trained to do what? They never made a bra small enough for me! A bunch of us went to the local ice cream parlor the night

I got my reward and I announced to everyone that I had gotten a bra! I guess I needed to have that strap across the back to finally come of age.

Throughout my grade school years, I had some friends whom I remember with lots of love. I always wanted to look like Jan. She had freckles, but they were better. Her hair was thicker and wavier. She never liked her teeth. But because I had a space between my teeth, I envied her teeth: the front ones were pushed in a little and the eye teeth were very prominent. She could whistle her S's. My friend Marsha and I have always been close, and we both have a space between our teeth. It's something special and, according to some, a sign of intelligence!

During early grade school years, I was always on the fringes of the "coolest" group, and I was also included in the group of girls who were smart and funloving. Later on, I needed to be included in the group with the "hangout house" when the boys were expected.

I was a friend to a lot of boys and girls from a very young age. However, my mother had always said, "Don't trust too many people." So I was afraid to have a best friend because that was a strong commitment and that friend might turn on me. So I tried to have a lot of friends, not just one best friend. I suffered with the social scene in some ways. I built up my wall by being friendly to everyone but not too close; that was my "protection."

When I was young, much of my wardrobe was handed down from my cousins, and beyond that, we were JCPenney shoppers. At Christmas, every box was from Penney's. My mother carried on the tradition of a big Christmas, no matter what, and it was wonderful. Even without a father and husband, we still had boxes and boxes of wonderful things under the tree—just we three women. Mother considered it important. There was always a doll and the matching Tycora sweater and socks as we got older. Christmas was always memorable and fun.

My father died from diabetes complications when I was in eighth grade. That was an extremely traumatic time in my life. Everyone was so concerned about my mother and my sister, but no one knew how special my father was to me. I didn't feel that anyone understood how really devastated I was when he died. I often think about the impact my father had on me, and my devastation in losing him. But God has given me a son who reminds me so much of my father and now I don't think about my father so much in sadness, but in joy and appreciation. Ironically, the long-range effect of my father's death was probably the most positive thing in my life. It made me a stronger person, a survivor.

My dad had always wanted me to go to the local Catholic girls' high school. We didn't have any money, but a priest friend of the family came to our aid with the tuition for the first couple of years of my high school education. I liked the environment at our all-girls' academy. I blossomed in a whole new group of people; I felt protected and smart enough to handle the courses. I chose the business curriculum because I wasn't going to college; there was no way we could swing it. But I got my better grades in history, English, biology, and algebra. I had a harder time with shorthand, typing, and bookkeeping. That's funny; I would have done well in college. I have great memories of high school because I knew that was the end of education for me.

After graduation it was the real world. I went to work. I was one of the first kids in our class to get a job through the school typing department. I worked part-time during the school year, and summers at a bedding supply company. And I got teased incessantly: "What are you doing? Testing mattresses?" But I got the best recommendation from that office manager. And it was read over the public address system at school. I felt so great! I'll never forget that letter; it was on marigold-colored stationery.

After graduation I got a job at the diocesan office, which didn't pay much. Mother and I were scouring the paper for a better long-term prospect, when we heard that IBM was testing and interviewing. By a fluke of fate, I had once babysat for the branch manager's family. However, I had scorched the popcorn, smelled the place up, and practically burned the house down, so I wasn't sure I'd get the job.

But I had to try. I flunked the test on the electric typewriter but I had the highest score in vocabulary and aptitude of all thirty applicants. And I got the job! So I had to decide between the diocesan office and IBM, which offered $300 a month and fabulous benefits. I chose IBM. What a fateful, wonderful decision! I started at IBM in July after graduation. I worked at IBM for ten years, and loved every minute of it.

To get to my first "big-time" work experience at IBM, I took the city bus. My mother laughed hysterically at me in spiked heels, a nice little dress, and gloves! She later said that watching me walk to the bus stop, at age 17, was more than she could handle.

And all the time I worked, my need for a college education was satisfied in two ways. I took evening courses in knitting, sewing, tailoring, art, history, English, Spanish, cooking and domestic engineering. I became a world traveller and IBM was very understanding when I needed more than my two weeks vacation for a long-awaited trip.

During those years at IBM, I hung out with all my friends at the college here in town. To this day, there are people who don't know that I never enrolled at that college. I went to all the parties and dances, all the Friday night mixers, all the balls, all the fraternity things—everything.

I dated extravagantly, but I fought romantic commitment for a long time. I wasn't the type who would scare a boy off. I was not at all serious; I always preferred to date the guys who were a little goofy. I felt safer! I could never be a real "bonus chick," I was the "filler chick," the fun one.

As for my appearance, I have had many different looks through the years, but one of my favorites was when I stopped being a blonde. I had been a blonde when I met my husband, Bill, at IBM in 1966. As I got to know him better, I just assumed he knew I was not a natural blonde. One night, he said, "How about going out for a pizza?" And I said, "I can't, I have to stay home and do my roots." He was floored. The man did not know that I colored my hair!

However, the blonde was difficult to keep up, and when I decided to go back to my natural color, the dye grabbed and came out way too dark. My friends didn't recognize me, but Bill, who had fallen in love with me as a blonde, really loved my naturally dark hair. I honestly feel that a lot of my self-image came from how he felt about me. I felt very attractive then. I knew he loved me. And because he was complimentary, I got instant feedback.

My favorite hairstyle was very dramatic. A friend commented that "it takes a lot of nerve to wear a center part when you have a space between your teeth!" My hair was shoulder-length in a full pageboy, parted in the center, with the sides pulled back over my ears. It was very severe with my dark ash-brown hair and distinctive features. My second favorite hairstyle was very casual, a short "wedge" cut with big fat bangs.

When I have haircuts that I really like, I project myself more—I seem to have more sparkle. A good appearance is so very important for women for self-image and self-esteem. I have never stayed with the same hairdo for too long, but I firmly believe I feel better about myself with a great haircut.

I believe in keeping up appearances and dressing appropriately for my age— not too young. I concentrate on looking good—for my sake, first of all, but also for my family's sake. If you have children, I think you do them a disservice if you start to look like you're worn down, don't know how to dress or take care of yourself. I think that's a bad message. You can always find nice things by creatively shopping and wardrobing. You don't need a ton of money to look good. And I think you cut your husband short if you don't try to look attractive for him. I see that as very important. Your family and friends respond positively to you if you look good, and they notice if you don't try.

I look more briefly in the mirror now than I used to; I try not to stand and study. I try not to notice the changes, because I don't want them to stop me from being friendly or from meeting new people. I don't want my age to stand in the way of my personality. So I do my routines a little faster, and I do not stand in front of the mirror and study my body too much! I put my clothes on real fast in the closet!

I have fun shopping skills, of which I am very proud. When I buy for myself, I always buy things on sale. It's like being naughty, shopping the sale racks on those rare occasions I shop for myself. I do the discount chain stores and the department store sale racks. I know exactly what works for my figure and I repeatedly bring things home that I haven't even tried on in the store.

And in my closets is all the stuff I have saved for years. Bill bought an outfit for me in New York at Bonwit Teller before we were married. I still have it: the hotpants, the tunic, the boots, and the gift box. And I have a beautiful polyester outfit in Chinese red, with bellbottom pants. And my lamé outfit. So I am a shopper, a bargain hunter, and a saver! You have to pity people like me with such a fixation. But I probably get more joy out of life than the people who toss everything away. I have had more fun for dress-up parties because of my shopping fetish! The only problem is, when I die, I want people to think of me as a happy shopper, not as a strange eccentric. Besides, by that time I figure I can donate it all to the local museum! I do sometimes threaten to throw things out, but I take them out of the closet and then put them back again; I cannot throw out my wonderful stuff. It's an idiosyncrasy that I am not willing to admit is strange.

Most of us believe that our appearance has played a big role in how we perceive ourselves. Mirror image and self-image are pretty much the same with me: what you see is what you get! I think others perceive me just the way I try to come across: friendly, easy to be around, and without airs. I don't intimidate people; I like to make them feel comfortable. That's my perception and that's the way I hope I am. I would be pretty surprised if someone called me "arrogant" or "superior," because I don't feel that way.

Yes, I am very happy with the person I am today. I wish I were more "up," but I don't think that is normal. In the roles of wife and mom to four kids, I sometimes feel put upon and I would like to be a little more lighthearted. But there are places in your life where you have to be serious and mine is in the family.

How am I going to deal with the aging process? I'm just going to get cuter and cuter! I'm just going to let it happen. I think that the aging process bothers me a whole lot less than the declining-health process. I don't like to think about how old I am or how many more years I have to be vital, but I don't have time to dwell on it because I have an agenda that just doesn't quit. I surround myself with fun people as a way to stay young. If you believe you're old, you are probably right.

I don't think of "retirement," just "investigating." I am a very curious person and always will be. I love making art, my watercolors. I hope to be painting, and painting, and painting until the day I die. Grandma Moses and me! I took up watercolors in mid-life and it has been such a joy. I have also had fun researching, designing, and supervising the building of our gazebo-studio room, as well as the pool, and deck area behind the house. That's another fun artistic outlet for me.

I recently started doing some art consulting to businesses in town, so my artistic endeavors continue to branch out. My youngest son was very complimentary to me just the other day. He said he was very proud of what I have accomplished. That was wonderful, because the kids have wondered why I never went to college; they thought maybe my grades weren't good enough!

My husband keeps my wardrobe current for me. He has a great knack for choosing things that work well for me. Special-occasion outfits for Mother's Day, my birthday, Christmas. He describes me, or what he would like, to the clerks when he's stuck. I assumed most husbands do the same thing, but I found out it's unusual. Husbands don't all do this and they sure don't understand their wife's style. My favorite outfits have been things that Bill has bought for me. Many of them are such classics, things that I can wear and wear and wear! It's been a fun part of our marriage. He knows me so well!

JAMIE, 19:
college student

When I was born, my mama was in labor for only five minutes! My grandmother tells the story of how she rushed my mama to the hospital. The nurses began to take mama upstairs as my grandma was filling out the registration information sheets. Then the nurse came back to tell her she was a grandmother. My grandma said, "No, not yet, I just brought my daughter here." And the nurse said, "I know and you are the grandmother of a brand new little girl!" So, born in five minutes, I have been said to be "quick, fast and in a hurry" ever since then. That's a very positive thing to me and that story tells you what kind of child I've always been!

I went to day care at the age of 2. My mother was getting ready to drop me off and see me into class as mothers do, but I said, "No, Mommy, I do it myself!" So I went into class by myself and had no problem. However, when my sister went to day care at age 2 she cried every day until she was 5, and she's seven years older than I am. That story also shows that I am strong, independent and on my own. I always wanted to do things by myself!

Growing up and going into high school I was skinny—very, very skinny. And I didn't have breasts like the other girls. They were all fully developed and I wasn't. In order to wear form-fitting clothes successfully you have to have a shape and I didn't, so I used to wear baggy jeans, baggy T-shirts and baggy sweats. I was already six feet tall and I played sports. I looked like a young boy and I didn't like that because I very much wanted to look like a woman and feel like a woman. Of course, I didn't because I didn't have any of the traits.

My grandmother hated my baggy clothes. She sews and she says the beauty of a garment is the way it's fitted to you. I didn't have any fitted garments because I didn't have any shape. So she took me to get some clothes. She always called me "Black Beauty." I am her Black Beauty! She gave me a little bit of self-confidence and I began to change.

My parents played both a positive and negative role in my self-image. My father's positive role was to instill hardworking ways. He works very hard. He has never missed a day at work. And I respect my mother—she is a loving mother. But they influenced me negatively in that they holler a lot. They are very aggressive. They also argue a lot. And being a child growing up, I did not like that at all. Even now, I don't like to argue. If I have to argue, then I have to walk away because I heard those arguments five or six times a day as a child, and it gets annoying. But they did push, and encourage and joke around. They were realistic about school—calm, cool and loving. My father is the type of person who doesn't care what you do, if you get a job that's fine. They are really pleasant these days.

During my grammar school years I attended St. Paul Lutheran School. I graduated in a class of twelve, so I was shy and churchgoing. As it turned out, I had to go to public high school because my sister was attending college but she hadn't gotten a scholarship, so my mother had to pay her tuition. For that reason I couldn't go to Walker Lutheran School which would have been the next level—the high school. I had a lot of growing up to do when I went to Austin High School.

It was a huge change. The kids were more experienced and advanced than we had been back at St. Paul. So, as a freshman, I was considered The Virgin at Austin. That goes to show you that everybody was having sex by that time! I kind of stood out. I was tall, I kept to myself, and I was quiet. My grade point average was 4.0. I did not like that school at first, because it was full of negativity and negative attention. The kids were told they wouldn't amount to anything! There were people in my freshman class that had kids. It was pretty bad.

Sophomore year I started getting into the swing of things. I was tired of being The Virgin and tired of being The Quiet Girl. I'm not a quiet person. I'm a gregarious person, so I decided to take a shot at it. I started to hang out and do what everyone else did.

My junior year I was a great basketball player, so I did the athletic thing and maintained my new popularity, too. I had been playing basketball since I was a kid, but my freshman year I had had major back surgery so I couldn't play. By my junior year, I kind of got more mature, hung out and just did my thing.

However, during those high school years and especially as a senior, I was nothing like I am now. I was just going with the flow of things and getting ready to graduate. My best memory of senior year was the prom. Prom was a big issue for us and, because all I ever did was wear sweats, everybody asked me what I was going to wear to the prom. Sweats? But I had a dress made and I looked absolutely beautiful. It fit me perfectly! It seemed like the day of the prom I had just grown breasts and a butt or grown bigger or something! I looked great and my date was so handsome! It was just like a dream come true. I felt like Cinderella. We had a limo and everything. So after that night everything just fell into place. Everything got better and better.

When I went away to college at the age of 16—which is very young—I went to Fort Smith, Arkansas, to a school called West Arkansas Junior College. I went there because I wanted to prep myself academically. I knew Austin High School had not prepared me for the college world. West Arkansas is #2 in academics in the country but it is also #1 in basketball, so I figured I couldn't go wrong. Checking it out, I discovered it was the place the other girls from Chicago had gone to get their degree and then had gone on to play major league ball. So, it was the best situation for me.

At age 16, I was ready to leave home! I left July 5, 1997, the day after the Fourth of July. I had to get away from my mom and dad. I had my own car and there was no curfew down there in Fort Smith. I just thought it was great. I thought I was very independent and on my own. But as I look back on it, my coach was right; I was very gullible and very naïve. I can see that now. People took advantage of me. I was considered to be rich. The people in Fort Smith are not materialistic and they thought I was this little rich girl when, in fact, I wasn't. I was from Chicago where "clothes are the thing" and I had a lot of clothes and a car. So people took advantage. They used my car all the time.

Then suddenly I had a boyfriend. My first love! And I thought we were going to get married and yada, yada. Well, it did not go like that at all! I began to see more and get a better vision of it as I got older and more mature. As a result, I became closer to God. I had grown up in a church-centered home. My freshman year in college I didn't go to church as much as I had been going; I went, but God was not the priority that He is now. I know when I have a problem that it's Him I seek out. It wasn't like that my freshman year. The more spiritual sense I got as a young adult, the wiser and more mature I got. Now, when things happen I just take it in, whereas I used to become really upset and furious with the whole thing. Now I just learn from my mistakes and I go on with it! As a young adult, I am a sponge—I am thirsty for wisdom. I love to talk to older people. They've been around longer than I have, so I'm pretty sure they have something to offer me. If I pay close enough attention, I can always learn and when people have something to say, they are wise enough not to waste the time in the telling.

For instance, when I got to high school, I had no one around saying, "Save your virginity, it's something beautiful." All I heard was, "You're a virgin? Goodness, you're so late!" I didn't have my sister to give advice. Of course, I wouldn't go to my mom! But I'm not making excuses; I made that decision myself.

My grandmother always gave me confidence and compliments. My first love, however, was more of a negative influence on me. He just played mental games with me and as I get older I can say I'm glad it happened that way, because now with every heartbreak I have, I know I no longer want to be with that person. Now I can just say "Goodbye, it's been nice meeting you." I've been through so much with relationships that I now know I don't need him, or him, or him. I can just sense it. And now I even actively look for the negatives, even though I know I'm not supposed to do that. I have the wisdom now, because I've had my feelings hurt.

On the positive side, my coach at West Arkansas was very, very, very supportive. He instilled in me how important it is to get a degree. How important it is to focus on academics. And be yourself. I have to thank him for that. Because here I am, a girl from Chicago; he didn't have to do that; he didn't have to take the time with me. He's one of the prophets in my life and I call him my white father, my white daddy!

I see myself today as very positive and very optimistic. I dream and I have dreams. Every night I pick out a star and say, "That star is shining down on me!" I have lots of goals. I want to play in the WNBA, I want to sing and act and be a model. These are huge dreams!

What I like about that is it sets me apart. These days, people of my generation don't dream anymore. I don't know why that is. Maybe it's because they don't believe they can do it. But all my life I have heard people say over and over again, "If you believe it, you can do it." At first, it sounds like crap, "Oh yeah, sure, I can!" But if you begin to visualize it and work for it, you can make it happen. The Bible says a man without a vision cannot prosper. I am really, really optimistic about my dreams. As I get older I focus more and more on what I want to do whereas before I was happy-go-lucky. I also try to avoid negative influences and friends because your friends show what kind of person you are. How can I have friends who are totally opposite of me? So I'm a little wiser and still thirsting for knowledge. I'm not as naïve or gullible. I'm very sure of myself, very certain. I'm 19 this year and a junior in college here in Chicago.

In terms of my self-image, it all goes back to prom night. I felt like a butterfly, I was floating all night. My date was tall—6'8"—and dark and handsome and I was tall—6'2"—and dark and beautiful in my perfectly beautiful dress that fit me perfectly. Everyone said I was beautiful and I felt beautiful, for the first time!

My freshman year in college my boyfriend would say certain things to put me down, like I guess the people around me thought that I thought that I was beautiful. I didn't really feel that way, I just thought I looked okay. Anyway, they started to mistreat me that way, "Oh, she thinks she's really beautiful!" That's what let me know they must have felt that way or they wouldn't have ever brought it up. So, I don't think I'm the most beautiful person in the world, but when I get my good clothes and make-up on I think I look pretty decent. Of course, I'm always really comfortable in my sweats!

I would describe myself, first of all, as very optimistic. And positive. I'm not a negative person at all. I am a dreamer and I have big aspirations. I'm also very, very goal oriented! In terms of my physical appearance, I see myself as a Black Beauty, as my grandmother always called me.

Of course, I look better now than when I was younger. As a child I was so skinny and my feet were so big. I really had to grow into my feet. Before my growth spurt, when I was short with big feet, I knew I was going to be tall, but I was kind of awkward. At that point, I saw myself as Olive Oyl. I wonder how I'll look as I get older, at 23 or so! As a whole, I see myself as a positive, religious, spiritual young lady.

My appearance is usually separate from my intellect and achievement. I'm usually in sweats, going to class, to work, or to basketball practice. When I'm dressed up I carry myself in a more positive way. But usually I don't take the time to look good everyday. I don't have the time. Sometimes I wonder if I should try to look better on a daily basis. I see the other girls walking around campus in their cute little capris, with their hair done, but I just don't have the time. I never have time! And it really takes time to curl your hair and do all that stuff! I just do sweats. It really shocks the guys because when they see me in sweats they think I'm just Jamie, but when I put on my good clothes they are like, "Wow!" They do one, two, three double-triple-takes! But on the other hand I am not here to impress anybody. I'm not here to judge a guy, but if I had a boyfriend, I'd want him to be okay with me in sweats because I'm not going to look glamorous every day. My recent ex-boyfriend always said, "Sweetie, you look beautiful dressed up and you look beautiful in sweats." I guess that's more me.

Others perceive me as very confident and doing my own thing. They say, "Jamie does what Jamie wants to do!" Some people have said I'm self-oriented, that I don't think about others. But that's not true. I have thought about others, but others have treated me badly. I have given my all. Gave 70 percent, got back 30 percent. Gave 80 percent, got back 20 percent. It's never been 50-50!

I have always had more guy friends than women friends. And with a certain guy who also played basketball I was always trying to pump him up. However, if I'd have pumped myself up I'd have been as uplifted he was! All I did was make somebody else happy. It used to be sad. I'm glad God has shown me the way. So now, instead of loving somebody else, I'm going to love myself. Now, Jamie needs to make Jamie happy! That's my thing. So, I'm calling the year 2000 Jamie's year. I'm going to think about me and do what I need to do for me.

So if other people perceive me as "Jamie is about Jamie," it's not the whole truth. Jamie is about Jamie, but Jamie is really about business first! I am not conceited, selfish, or arrogant in the way they think. I will help someone if I can, but only as long as it doesn't deter me in my goals. And that person must do something in return for me. I simply can't do what I used to do because it was to my own detriment.

I am very happy with the person I am today, although I do have a big change I would like to make. My first love was not a positive influence; ours was not a great relationship. And I want to be in a good relationship so badly! But I am not a patient person at all. If I had patience, I'd be blessed. But I'm so impatient it's ridiculous and especially with relationships. I'm tired of being alone. But I don't want the wrong person. If I could be patient, I know I'd be better off.

The thing that's kept me on track all these years is that I've always wanted to play professional basketball. And I knew I had to get good grades—a good G.P.A.—and I've always liked school. School was never a problem for me. I've always been impatient waiting for school to start. Classes have always been easy for me. I've never had a class that was truly academically challenging—well, one! I'm really a very smart young lady and I can compete comfortably but I have just never done the homework. I never did or learned to do homework. In grammar school we did all our work in class and in high school it was so bad they didn't give homework. So I had a hard time getting used to the hang of things. That's part of maturity. Basketball was all I ever wanted to do and I knew I had to go to school. Fortunately, I loved school!

Getting through high school without having a baby like most of my classmates, is directly related to my hopes and dreams! Growing up on the west side of Chicago, living the life I have and experiencing the things I have, I realized people can be better off. I've watched other people, as well as their moms and dads, and I concluded there was a better way. I don't want to struggle with my child. And I don't want her to struggle like my parents did. My husband-to-be and I will want the best for our child. It may sound materialistic, but she's going to have a Benz when she's 16 and go to Florida on spring break. Having a baby at a young age is just stupidity. I'm not saying I'm not having sex and I can even understand one mistake, but with two or three kids you get on welfare and you never get off. It's just a cycle.

I want to start my kids off on the right foot. Even if I had a child now and didn't graduate from college, where would I get the money for my child to go to college? I have to think about that. I don't want my child to ever have to worry about anything. I will not have children until they can have the best. It all goes back to dreams and aspirations. Many girls get a boyfriend who buys them a couple pairs of shoes and pays for getting her hair done. She thinks that's the ideal world. But to me that's nothing because I know what I want to be. Jamie! Having a child whose father buys you new shoes every other week is not the world of my dreams. Maybe it's fine for them, but not for me. By the time we were seniors in high school, we had girls in our class who were on their second child! That's really sad. And the dropouts? We started with about 850 freshmen and we graduated 101! Austin is not a good place. The school just got off academic probation this year—from 1993 to 2000! The kids didn't have goals. But it all goes back to the parents. If they don't set up positive role models and goal models, the kids don't follow through. But that's what my mother did. When people asked why she sent me to Austin instead of the Lutheran high school, she always said I was strong enough to achieve anywhere and that in our house I was expected to achieve. Most of the kids I grew up with didn't have the kind of parents I had. Their parents were often on drugs and alcohol. Their parents didn't look out for them. They had to take care of themselves. But I'm a girl from the 'hood, so people could see that I did it and if I could do it, they could do it! But it's a big responsibility to be that kind of role model, too! These days eighth graders have no greater goal than just to graduate from eighth grade. And some of them have babies already!

My mother had had two years of college but she dropped out to have my sister and she never went back. My father didn't even go to college. He worked. In a steel mill. It goes back to the old thing: men got jobs. My sister, my only sibling, was my role model for completing a college degree.

She graduated from Jackson State University in Mississippi in speech and dramatic arts. She now works for SmithKline Beecham. They have just moved her from Atlanta back here to Chicago. She's a manager. She's applying for graduate school now to get her master's. Her dream is to buy a theatre. She speaks really well. When she speaks, you get the chills!

There are four black girls on our university basketball team. Two are from Addison. One is from Country Club Hills. And I am from the west side. I'm so different from them! When we are in airports while travelling with the team, they would rather be home, but I feel I am really blessed to be travelling. We're going to Europe this summer! It's just a blessing to me! Milan, Paris and Rome. The NBA and WNBA play in Europe over the summer, so I'm sure we'll meet some people and there will be some people looking at us—professionally!

J A N E, 47:
creative writer: advertising

My earliest mental images of myself are related to my mother, the person I was around most as a child. I judged myself by her; I wanted to be as pretty as she was. My mother always looked very pulled-together and well-groomed. I loved playing dress-up in her clothes and shoes. I also judged myself by my friends, and if they had pretty hair or a pretty dress, I probably copied them.

From family photographs I realize I was a funny-looking little kid in my fancy outfits. As the first girl in the family after many, many boys, I had aunts and grandmothers happily sewing for me. I finally learned to make my own clothes from one of my aunts and from sewing classes in school. So this appearance thing has been important and continual throughout my life and I am very much aware of it.

Several years ago I went to a women's seminar, where we were asked to bring photographs of ourselves as a child, little girl, teenager, and young adult. I hadn't seen a lot of these pictures in years, and I remember thinking, "God, what a little Kewpie doll I was!" I had golden ringlets that my mother played with all the time and I always wore fancy little dresses. I guess I got my first sense of myself as my mother's little doll because she was always fussing with me. In fact, I had a thing with my hair until I was married; I worried about my hair all the time. It had to be done perfectly.

Obviously my mother had been obsessed with my hair. She was always curling it and fixing it. I was probably the little girl everyone else hated: so cute and with such pretty ringlets. My hair and my overall appearance was really important to my mother. And it was important to me. Even as a child, I was very aware of how my hair looked all the time.

One day a friend got hold of a pair of scissors and cut off all my locks because she thought they were funny-looking. When I came home, my mother went absolutely crazy, forbidding me to play with the girl again. I didn't understand what the big deal was because I was finally liberated from those curls. And I didn't know why I was forbidden to play with that girl just because she had cut off all my hair.

I was a young adult in the 1960s and my hairstyles, which required setting on brush rollers all the time, were not conducive to romance or married life, so I had to find other ways to deal with my hair. It all started when I began regular exercise workouts, because playing with my hair took too much time. At that point I tried a perm with a wash-and-wear style. Now, I keep my hair well-cut but very simply styled.

There are all kinds of traumatic experiences around my hair because a "bad hair day" usually ruined my life. I got my first perm as a young child, and even though my mother took me to a beauty shop, they didn't know what to do with my very fine hair. My hair literally came off on the perm rods as they were unrolling it. Mother contemplated a lawsuit but never went through with it, and then began giving me home perms (which were not an improvement).

When I was a youngster, this fussing over my appearance was constant; I never wanted to ruin my hair or my outfit. Obviously, I was never encouraged to go into sports or messy activities because that was contrary to looking proper. So I was never very active, which has been a detriment all my life. I was not conscious of avoiding getting messed up; it was so ingrained that I didn't even think about it. Mostly, I just didn't do much.

At 10, 11, and 12 years of age, we neighborhood girls spent our time dressing our dolls and putting on stage shows and fashion shows. Dragging our mothers' clothes and shoes, we would adjourn to someone's basement or attic to play fashion show. The parents of one friend owned an unoccupied storefront building, so we had a big space in which to put on musical shows using the song books from the Hit Parade radio program.

Teenage and high school years were terrible times for me. I didn't see myself as particularly attractive in high school, but it was all my best friend's fault because she was beautiful and got all the attention! At sock hops and dances she always got asked to dance. And even though she never ended up dating anybody, I attributed my bad feelings about myself to her. In reality I just didn't have it together and lived in her shadow. We took sewing class together in high school and our last names were similar, so people confused us because we did all the same activities. Her clothes were always perfectly turned out. She got the lead parts in all the plays. One of those people. Every school has that same girl. You just hope that she's not your friend!

I never had a bad self-image, but I was never really happy with the way I looked. When, as an adult, I started working out, I finally developed a very high comfort level with who I was and what I looked like. And I was also able to improve my appearance in ways I had always wanted but didn't think were possible. Up to that point I was never overweight but never happy with the way my body looked; I wanted to lose this or change that. Exercise really helped me realize I could do something about my body if I wanted to. That was a real turning point. And then, too, taking dance classes as an adult helped me to develop a sense of poise and grace and become more comfortable with the way I moved.

Also I finally learned that body consciousness was okay. A Catholic education had taught us that our body was never supposed to be important; we were never supposed to be comfortable with it or show it off because that was bad. I was in my early 30s before I learned that if I looked good in something, then I should wear it because it enhanced me. It was not shameful and didn't make me look like a hussy or loose woman. That lesson was important to me because it was the first time I felt really good about myself. Not only was I totally happy with my body but, with my great new perm, I didn't have to worry about my hair anymore. It was a totally liberating experience that solved all kinds of problems.

For many years I have worked in the advertising business, where appearance is very important and where you are surrounded by people who constantly measure you, give you points, or think poorly of you based on what you wear or how your hair looks. In my young adulthood, I felt that I could not comfortably wear theatrical or provocative clothes, but now I feel differently. My experience in the advertising business, with its performance aspects and "show biz" atmosphere, taught me that the people whose work gets noticed and who get promoted were not afraid to call attention to themselves with an interesting combination of looks, actions, and skills.

So at the point where I was getting comfortable with my body and myself, I also began to experiment with my appearance. And suddenly, when I walked into a conference or gave a presentation, I noticed that I was perceived differently: I was somebody who had it all together and who commanded attention. In that business it is very important to walk into a room and command attention immediately, because when you have everyone's respect, they want to hear what you have to say. The premise is that if you look creative, you obviously think that way. Fortunately my experiments in appearance brought it all together for me because I am a quiet person whose personality does not command attention. Dressing was the best way for me to get attention and, within certain parameters, it worked, which was very helpful.

Later on, however, when I worked for a woman supervisor, my appearance and body confidence didn't serve me as well with her. There was really nothing wrong with her appearance, but the fact that I looked so good bothered her a lot. I wasn't aware of it then or I would have done something about it. I didn't find out until later when a male co-worker said, "You really annoy Anita! The clothes you wear, and the way you look really gets under her skin." I thought my performance was bothering her, but it had nothing to do with that: she thought I was trying to be too glamorous, trying to get too much attention. So it works both ways even in the creative business.

I have been told that I intimidated people, though I didn't realize it at the time. When I told a gay male friend that I had very few close women friends, his response was, "Well, that's easy to see. You are really an intimidating person!" He insisted that I probably scare the pants off most people. People do tell me that I appear aloof, although I don't see myself that way. What others see as aloofness, I see as quiet and shy behavior, so I don't think most of us understand that our appearance and manner can intimidate others.

I never felt that I looked really good even during the time when I felt the best about myself and was intimidating to others. Now, however, I am comfortable with this package that is me—even with 15 extra pounds. I'm not beating myself up over it, but I still don't think it's the best I can be. Are there women who just wake up every day and say, "I feel great and I look great"?

People have probably said that I paid too much attention to my appearance; however, I still get compliments about the way I put things together even though I don't spend a lot of time at it. I probably appear as if I spend more time than I do because other people perceive wardrobe coordination as a time-consuming practice. It's really just a matter of seeing the right accessory. And then, too, I have my share of things in the closet that don't work.

I probably will always subscribe to a wide selection of fashion magazines to inspire creativity, new combinations, or ways of looking at things. That is a talent that applies to my entire life, not just my clothes. To be creative, I need to expose myself to new ideas in words as well as pictures. I need to open up my horizons and be receptive, be a sponge, appreciate the whole spectrum of life, art, etc. Everything I see or read becomes part of the memory bank for my creative work. Fashion is the same. If I am aware of a new look, I can use pieces of it to look current and personalized.

I'm pretty happy with the person I am today. As for the aging process, the vain part of me says go for a face-lift, but the practical side says, "What if the surgeon strikes a nerve?" In June I went to a high school reunion. When the invitation went out in April, one of my friends, who had been thinking about plastic surgery, immediately went out and had a mini-face-lift. That just blew me away. I consider myself to be a fairly vain person, but I don't feel insecure with people I went to school with and have known for years. She looked great, but she was the only one who ran out and did that. It wasn't really obvious, but I knew it was more than just a new moisturizer! The truth is, your hands show your age sooner or later and you can't hide them. Your hands actually play up the fact that you've had your face done.

Keeping yourself looking current, however, can change how you see yourself in relation to your age. Even grey hair looks great in a current style with an up-to-date wardrobe. Many women my age look and feel and act much older than I feel or think of myself. Your sense of age has a lot to do with the things life hands you, but still your attitude is very important. An acquaintance, who is my age, talks about herself as a grandmother and recent widow and has a double dose of an old self-image. She has talked herself into it, too. On the other hand, my mother thinks other people her age look older than she does! It's all in the mind.

JANET, 48:

musician, music teacher

There's a Norman Rockwell print that sums up my feelings about myself. It's a picture of a little girl about 9 years old with pigtails, a black eye, and bruised and skinned knees, sitting outside the principal's office. Her hair is all messed up, but she's got a smug expression on her face and a little twinkle in her eye. She's obviously been in a fight but she has a look of real self-satisfaction. Through the doorway is the principal and a teacher discussing what's going to happen to her now that she's been a bad girl. Initially the print grabbed my eye because I really looked very much like that at the same age and it represents the tomboyish and confrontational side of me. But the best part is that the picture is called "The Winner"! From this vantage point in life, I am also a winner—bruised and battered, but a winner.

The picture reflects, even more than my childhood, the bad time after the divorce from my first husband, John. I spent five years reorganizing my retail business and adjusting first to my new single life and then to life with my second husband, Jim, but mostly I was resolving all kinds of frightening issues. There were all kinds of personal and legal issues with John while terminating the marriage and the business. But finding this print last year was a real highlight! It expresses visually some very strong feelings of worth in overcoming all odds. This has been a central theme of my life.

As a little girl, I was very boyish and prided myself on having only boys as best friends. There was Butch next door and Stevie, whom I adored, in the other side of the duplex. There was also Roger, who lived around the corner, and Larry and Johnny. Those were my buddies. The girls who lived on the other end of the block did really stupid little girlie things. I preferred to get out my trucks or get on my cowboy clothes and make Indian teepees and soldiers' forts with the boys.

Butch had a mean streak, though; he was a bully who used to get a little bit rough and sometimes tear my clothes. One winter day, my dad saw

Butch and Larry push me down on the ice rink and wash my face with snow. The snow was scratchy and hurt my face, and I remember feeling very scared and trapped. When Dad yelled at the boys, they went running and I came home crying. Then Dad gave me a lesson in self-defense. He taught me how to turn around and kick the bully in the shin with my heel. I remember using that technique one day when Larry took my arm and twisted it up behind my back. I whacked him in the shin so hard that he cried!

So I was a tomboy. I saw myself that way and I identified with my dad. I was 9 or 10 when the family began to be concerned because I walked like a boy with great big strides. My sister Lois decided it was time that I learned to "address my femininity." Lois, who was older by 12 years, was always very good to me and had a major influence on me all through my childhood. She took me aside one day, saying we were going to learn to walk with good posture. Together we practiced walking with books on our heads to change my gait into something a little more feminine and graceful. She also bought me a manicure set and did my nails. She started reading me stories about Cinderella and encouraged me to play with dolls. All these things were intended to feminize me. Lois brought me around from excessive boyishness, and I learned to enjoy those times with her.

In seventh grade, Lois and my mother gave me my first permanent. In spite of their best efforts, it turned out all fuzzy and frizzy and I felt like an absolute geek. Sometimes I didn't like the clothes my mother bought for me; even though I thought I was very much a tomboy up until seventh grade, I didn't want to wear anything mannish with pads in the shoulders.

My parents were both very influential in my life and in the formation of my self-concept, but in very different ways. From early on, I bonded with Dad and felt really close and emotionally safe with him. Mother was the disciplinarian. She spanked hard with the hairbrush on the bare bottom. I used to get spanked practically every day, as I recall. And if I sassed her back it was Fels Naphtha soap scraped on the teeth. She was really strict, and if she got angry there was a lot of denial of her love. She wouldn't speak to me. One time she pretended she was packing her suitcase to leave for good. She had ways of really making a point!

I went to elementary school at St. Mary's with the Polish Catholic nuns. It always reminds me of "Do Patent Leather Shoes Really Reflect Up?" Both the school and the nuns were very influential in my childhood. The attitudes were typical of the 1950s and a strict upbringing. There was a lot of emphasis on sin and not thinking about "it" (sex). I had an underlying anxiety about being in school. The nuns were very sweet and motherly in the earliest grades, but the fourth-grade sister was real stern and grouchy. She hit me. As we got older, my classmates and I learned to turn the tables on the teachers. We organized classroom pranks like group book drops to upset the elderly nuns who could no longer control us, and we constantly pestered the younger nuns with "theological" questions like, "How could the Virgin Mary get pregnant by a bird?" We loved to peek over the convent fence on laundry days to see what the nuns wore underneath their habits.

By eighth grade we were already anticipating going to the Academy, the all-girls' high school. I was really looking forward to the uniforms and the whole grownup scene, but the downside was that Mother forbade me to pal around with my old grade-school friends anymore! So starting off at the Academy at age 14, that gawky age, was very hard. My hair began to fall out. Another classmate, Kris, used to pull out her eyebrows. We were all going through that kind of stuff. I didn't really have any friends. I had never been outgoing; I used to wait for people to call me. Of course, nobody ever did, so I got depressed and cried a lot. When my hair started falling out behind my ears, I had to wear gooky ointment that plastered my hair down flat. I felt like such an outcast. I used to break down and cry at my piano lessons with Sister Laurent.

During that time, Mother was actually pretty supportive when I came home and cried about that stuff, but she also pushed me to be more social. One winter day she looked out the window and said, "There's somebody over there ice skating. Just get on your warm clothes and skates and go over there and make friends with that person." I got my stuff on and trudged over there thinking I was going to have to make friends with a total stranger. When I finally got over there, I heaved a sigh of relief because it was my neighbor Colleen! When I got back home all happy, Mother said, "Now see, you had a good time. What was she like?" "It was Colleen, Mom!"

I always liked being alone as a kid and I still do. Mother always thought something was wrong with me because I often sought out isolation. She made me think I wasn't normal, but it was what I liked to do.

In high school, one of the things that contributed so much to my "inferiority complex" was my crooked teeth. My canine teeth protruded beyond my two front teeth. I was so self-conscious, that I actually covered my mouth when I laughed. And to top it all off, the kids in grade school nicknamed me "Fang"! The nasty kids did that; they said it in front of other people. I was so embarrassed and it contributed to the feeling that I wasn't as good as other people and that I wasn't pretty.

When I expressed my negative feelings to my parents, they had me see a dentist. I was absolutely elated that maybe I could get my teeth fixed. Braces would have made a major difference in my self-image, but they were too much money. Dad said no; I cried. Mother said "But that's your personal trait." It didn't get any better; I hated my "trait" all through high school. I suppose everybody has something they dislike about themselves and then focus on. My thing was my teeth.

To compensate, I tried to play up my hair. I let my hair grow with the idea that by the time we graduated, I would have the longest hair of anyone in our high school. By the time my hair got nice and long, it had become my new trait. When the movie "South Pacific" came out, I started wearing my hair like Tup-Tim, pulled straight back and tight, the hot new look.

Sophomore year I got involved in the school musicals and started feeling a little more confident despite my teeth. I started going out on dates, but I was still very introverted. I never ventured to run for a class office or a club office. By that time, though, I was starting to make friends and do things with other people. A group of us went to the Friday night dances at the boys' high school; that started a cohesiveness among us. The group fluctuated all the time, but Kris, Marsha, Maureen, and I started to be a foursome of sorts. There were other kids in homeroom, too, whom I started being more comfortable with and then I branched out from there.

There were lots of boys I wanted to notice me but who didn't. Back then girls did not make the first move. They waited for it to happen and hoped it would be the boy they liked. I wasn't allowed to date until I was a sophomore when my first date was with Bill. Then I went out with Peter once or twice and he was my new heartthrob. I began to feel a little more confident about myself. By the time I was 16 and driving Dad's car to school, all the boys would be waiting for us after the dismissal bell. My favorite boyfriend at that time was Bob who used to leave little notes on my windshield wipers addressed to "Princess."

As my figure developed, clothes became an avenue to feeling pretty. Mother always liked beautiful clothes, so she was very supportive of how I looked and bought me beautiful things to wear for special occasions because we wore uniforms to school. I was lucky for that. I got into the habit of having a pair of shoes for every outfit. If there was a formal dance coming up we automatically went shopping.

I loved a green plaid taffeta dress with puffy sleeves and a skirt that twirled. I also had a navy skirt with a pink poodle applique and a coordinating blouse that was pink with a navy poodle. I wore that outfit with many, many crinolines—the thing back then.

I often babysat for my aunt, Jeanette, who was another important role model in terms of appearance. Jeanette had wonderful clothes and with her permission I had great fun going up to her bedroom and trying on her things. I loved to put on her makeup, clothes, jewelry, and shoes and check myself out in the mirror for hours. Later on, when I was dating, she sometimes let me wear her clothes for special occasions because we wore the same size. It was always a special treat to pick something from Jeanette's wardrobe to wear to homecoming or a prom.

We didn't have a lot of money but appearance things were attended to. Mother didn't work except to take care of Grampa and Gramma, who was bedridden. I know Grampa paid Mother something and I know she used a lot of that money for my clothes. Although later on she also just gave me her permission to charge at her favorite stores. By then I could go shopping and pick out clothes myself—whatever I wanted and whenever I wanted. Fortunately, I never went overboard; I was careful.

However, there is one bad story about Mother that stands out in my memory. Old enough to babysit, I must have been 13 by then. I wanted to save enough money and to pick out something for myself and buy it with my own money. At the local department store I had spotted a dress in a printed voile fabric of dark brown, purple, and green. It had a high neck with lace trim, puffy sleeves, and a bow that tied in the back. It was featured on a mannequin and I thought it was a very beautiful dress. It appealed to my 13-year-old taste. And it was the first time I had ever asserted myself to pick out something on my own. I didn't tell anyone about the dress. It was going to be a surprise.

I had talked to the saleswoman who was very nice to me. She knew I loved the dress. Promising to keep the dress for me, she encouraged me to save my money. In a couple of weeks when I had the $15, which was a lot of money in the 1950s, I took the bus downtown and bought the dress. When I came home with the box I said, "Mother, I have a surprise for you. I want to show you what I bought." I was so excited. I put the box on the bed, opened it up, and took out the dress. And Mother asked, "You bought that dress? Why would you pick that dress?" And I said, "Well, I like it. It's a pretty dress. I've liked it for a long time and I've been saving my money to buy it. Don't you like it?" Mother kept saying, "Oh, Janet! How could you pick out something like that?"

I had been very proud that I saved my money to buy the dress. And for some reason the incident became a really traumatic thing for me. Mother really put down my taste for picking out that dress and insisted that I return it. I didn't want to and I begged her, "Don't make me take this dress back. There's nothing wrong with it. I love this dress." I went through such agony over that dress. It represented not just a personal choice but doing something on my own, which was very important. Well, she insisted that I bring the dress back. I was crying so hard that I had to wear sunglasses during the bus ride back to the store. I was so embarrassed, but I could not stop crying.

Before returning the dress, I went to see Dad at work. When he saw how upset I was he took me into a back room for a private discussion. Sobbing and barely able to talk, I opened the box. I explained how Mother was making me return the dress, which I had bought all by myself. "Look, it's a pretty dress; I don't want to take it back." He said "I don't see anything wrong with it." But he also said I had to bring it back. To this day, I really feel he should have called her and said, "Florence, let her keep that dress. She's very proud of it. It's a good thing that she did. You shouldn't make her bring it back." But he didn't say anything to Mother. I had to bring the dress back and I remember how sad the saleslady was, too. She felt so bad; I felt so bad. I was still crying. From this vantage point I believe Mother was worried about what people would think. She didn't think the dress was quite what she would have picked out and that people would ultimately get a bad impression of her, not me.

I haven't really resolved my personal image, in terms of one consistent look. I still experiment and give in to my whims and fancies, so I have a variety of styles that I pick according to my mood or the situation. I have come away from a too-perfect look, however. I don't want to be quite so perfect anymore. I used to be a fanatic about my hair. If it wasn't perfect I was miserable all day.

When I had my own interior design shop, I chose to play the game of looking like an authority. I tried to look chic, keeping my hair really short. I bought clothes that were neither ultra feminine nor ultra masculine. As a woman in business I wore a lot of black but always with a flower on my lapel or a lace hankie in my pocket. Sometimes I looked very arty and sometimes very businesslike; it depended on my schedule for the day. So there was a mix of looks that I used successfully.

I have always been careful not to intimidate clients, so when I relocated my interior design business to a town of about 5,000, I felt I had to change my look. I had been working in the city with more educated, well-travelled people. This is a more blue-collar community and to reach them I cannot look too high-tech. So I dressed down but "up." I had to buy different kinds of clothes and change my appearance somewhat. I had to be a little more conservative or dressed-up-casual, not too severe or too arty.

At this point, I am no longer in the design business. I have let that go while focusing more on peace and quiet, music, and creativity in a private way. I keep four little hens and I put on concerts in my home. Now I feel even freer to dress like the local eccentric. I revel in that. And now that I have been here in town for a while, I can pull out some of my arty clothes again and wear them if I feel like it. And I don't have to be perfect when I go to the grocery store. If I want to go in jeans with mud on my knees from kneeling in the garden, that's okay. I don't care—it's honest work.

These days I teach piano and organ and avoid any clothes that look too teacher-like or severe. Sometimes I look in the mirror and scare myself because I see my mother. I don't want to take on the image of her in my mind—that stern and self-righteous look. I want to look more casual and approachable. For dealing with my very young students I dress casually, often wearing jeans and boots, a big sweater and loopy earrings. With the adults I dress up a little bit more. It depends.

I feel comfortable about the way I look now as long as I have clothes on. My husband, Jim, is very supportive. He thinks my body is great even when I'm not wearing clothes. He tells me I have the body of a 19-year-old, but maybe he's just not seeing too well these days!

It's a matter of adjusting to my appearance now. I'm getting lots of "silver" hair, which I like. It's fun to do things with it. I've got my hair long again, after having it short for many years. It will probably be short again some time soon. Currently I'm experimenting to develop a new sense of contentment with the changes I have to deal with at this age. Maybe I'll have a face-lift sometime if I can save a few bucks and have a few things taken care of in the eye area. I wouldn't want to get rid of all my wrinkles. I like the laugh lines around the eyes, but I don't like the furrow, the frown lines between the eyebrows.

I expect that I will always feel young. And I will enjoy associating with young people as well as working with old people. I don't think that I should try to look too young; looking like a teenager is not the way to go. I think you should play up your assets whatever they are. And if you can change things you don't like, go for it. People should be open to try new things.

I never had a sense of having a home life in my first marriage, and now I just really revel in my home and my home life. I enjoyed being an entrepreneur, making my own way, and being my own boss, definitely. But selling some land that I inherited and investing in a duplex on the bay, and restoring an 1886 brick schoolhouse and a 1974-vintage pontoon houseboat satisfies that need to challenge myself and remain in the business world. I get enough satisfaction and pleasure out of that. I suppose it goes back to my picture of "The Winner." The duplex satisfies the need to secure my own future and do something new; it was a good move. The houseboat and the schoolhouse are creative ventures with income potential, but mostly they are outlets to channel skills I have learned and to keep the adventures going. Teaching music to adults and children on a one-to-one basis satisfies the private creative thing focused on individuals. Directing our community chorus has now opened up another world. I really enjoy my new lifestyle.

I have had my teeth straightened as an adult, before I left my first marriage, and I love my new teeth. I wore braces for 3 1/2 years, taking them off a week before I met Jim. Having the braces on never bothered me; I felt wonderful wearing them. Far from making me self-conscious, they made a major difference in my self-image. And I know that I put out more positive vibes and a sense of confidence that make me more approachable.

Had that been done years ago, I wonder if things might have been different in my life. I have a feeling that I would have made some different choices, met other kinds of men, been a little more bold and I wouldn't have settled for what I did in my first marriage. I have that feeling. But all's well that ends well. And things are really very well.

The major thing I wish I could change about myself is my unreasonable fear of public performance, getting up in front of people to perform solo on the piano or organ. The reason I'm so disgusted with myself is because I really have something to share in my music. But I can't. Well, I can but my best work is not done in public. I wish I could play in public like I do when I'm alone but it just doesn't happen that way. And I don't know how to get over it. Maybe some day I will figure it out. It goes way back. It's in the gut. It's powerful. I am simply too afraid to go out and perform solo. When I was a little girl people would say, "there's nothing she can't play." In my mind I knew better but I thought they expected me to play everything. I thought they expected perfection. I don't know if it is fear of making a mistake or a self-conscious reaction.

Last year I went to a hypno-therapist to figure out what was behind all this panic and fear of solo performance. It took me a long time to work through those feelings. I recently performed solo at one of my student recitals; I got through it and I didn't die! I now use breathing and relaxation techniques and beta-blockers if necessary. But I learned that I can do it and get control of most of the fear!

POSTSCRIPT: At age 55 I had a face-lift! It has restored my "can do" attitude at a time when it was beginning to slip.

JENNIFER, 21:
college student

The first memory I have of my appearance dates back to kindergarten. In preparation for a family trip to Florida, my mom had cut my hair in a kind of bowl cut. When we returned from the trip, I went back to school expecting people to notice my haircut because no one there had seen it. I got many different reactions: "You got a haircut." "It looks good." "I don't like it." I went on playing and soon forgot about it, but I remember being cognizant of the fact that something was different about me and that I expected people to respond.

Childhood incidents that contributed to my self-image were all very positive. My mom always told me, "You're so cute. You're so nice, so sweet. You look so nice in that outfit." And my dad did the same. There were a lot of positive affirmations about my looks and my personality. I grew up with high self-esteem; I never worried about how I looked.

Although my mom was always overweight, she was, and still is, very comfortable with her size. She likes being a heavier woman. She was a size 8 when she was married, but she says she feels healthier and better about herself when she weighs more. My mom is an excellent role model for a larger woman who is comfortable in her body. As a result, I have never had a fear of being overweight; it was never a negative thing. I still don't fear it.

On the other hand, my mom didn't allow me to eat junk food. I always had healthy home-cooked meals, and I was always allowed a treat as long as I had eaten something healthy first. It was more of a health issue than a reaction to weight gain. The rule was, "Eat when you're hungry," so I could eat pretty much when I wanted, but she kept an eye on me to make sure I ate the right things because I had a sweet tooth.

As a child, I was very talkative and very inquisitive and I was made to feel sensitive about it because, although my parents never stifled those qualities, relatives and teachers often did. That made me unsure about the proper way to act and I am still struggling to develop an appropriate assertiveness.

I have an older sister, and the key factor in our upbringing was that my mom never allowed us to attack each other physically or verbally. I had a gap between my teeth and my sister's two front teeth just barely crossed over. We had an ongoing war: I called her Miss Crossover Teeth; she called me Miss Gap Between Her Teeth. My mom always interfered in these wars and told us that each was the only sibling the other had, and that once our parents were dead no one would ever be able to love us as well as we could love each other because we were flesh and blood. She believed the whole world might rip us apart during our lifetime, so why would we do it to each other? She never allowed us to attack each other over our looks, our clothes, or our girlfriends and boyfriends.

I think that was so important because my mom's sister raised her family very differently. Her four girls grew up being able to go at each other's throats and make fun of each other and their friends. As a result, they all have low self-esteem. Even as grown women, they attack each other from all angles. If one eats a piece of pie, the others will say, "Leave some for us, fatso!"

When I was about 14, one of these cousins started making fun of my eyebrows. I had never thought about my eyebrows until she began calling me O.B. (like the tampon), which meant one-brow. She made me so self-conscious about my eyebrows growing right across the bridge of my nose that I went out and had my eyebrows waxed. It was a horrific experience and such an unnatural thing for me to do, especially at that age. I saw the immense amount of pressure that can be put on someone; it made a powerful impression on me because in my family we just didn't do that.

In my early years in elementary school, I was tracked as a gifted student. I went through all the excelled classes and the special gifted program. I won the junior high chess tournament, all the math awards, spelling bees, and science fair projects, all of which built up my self-esteem. I wasn't concerned with my looks or popularity.

However, between eighth and ninth grade, all that changed drastically when I became aware that girls were wearing makeup, shaving their legs, and starting to date boys. I still had straight hair and wasn't very feminine. I thought I'd better get with it, so I went through a big process to feminize myself.

My role model was a beautiful cheerleader who was in high school when I was in eighth grade. I wanted to look like her so I got my hair done like hers; I wanted to be like her so I tried out for cheerleading squad and made it. And that was the beginning of a real tragedy in my life because once I became more mature looking and gained popularity, I started adapting to what I thought was the appropriate lifestyle: flirting and dating football players. It was as if in this world I couldn't be both pretty and smart.

As I got prettier, I became more concerned with being popular and less concerned with achieving academically. I knew I was smart and could get by with at least a B, so I never put in the time or effort. I started down that road of my own choice—I chose to be popular and beautiful—but everyone agreed that it was a nice role for me. It fit. I was "the pretty one," so I should be popular and should date boys.

My sister, who was two years older and in high school at the time, had always been very smart and never got sidetracked the way I did with notions of popularity and beauty. She never had much of a social life or many dates. My parents saw her as "the smart one" because, although she is very attractive, she never bothered to enhance her looks.

My parents accepted and even promoted these roles for my sister and me. Once I became a cheerleader, that became my new identity in everyone's mind. They acted as if I had blossomed into my real personhood as a flighty, ditsy, good-looking cheerleader. And that became what everyone expected of me. My teachers expected less of me academically, my social circle expected more of my time. I found it impossible to deviate from that path. I was conscious that I was trapped. I was still going to the advanced placement classes, but I was no longer taken seriously. I could no longer assert myself academically once I had asserted myself as a teen icon.

From the time I realized I didn't want to stay in that role, I've been fighting an uphill battle with everyone, including my family, to prove that there is something else to me. Even now when my sister and I go to family dinners, everyone asks my sister questions about the president's new communications bill or about the capital of Ghana. Even though I'm a political science major they ask me who I'm dating, and whether or not I've lost weight or changed my hair. It really frustrates me; it's very painful.

I realize that my community—a blue-collar Midwest manufacturing town—expected nothing more of females than marriage, kids, and a cosmetology career. When I wanted to do something other than that—go to college and get an education—it was considered ludicrous. Because I was pretty, I was supposed to just trap a man and "settle down." Because my sister didn't play up her looks, everyone thought she might have to go to college because she might not get married. While I struggled desperately to find what I thought would be an appropriate professional career path in public relations or television broadcasting and to go to an out-of-state college, my high school counselor arranged several home economics mentorships for me and advised me to go to the community college.

Although I finally succeeded in going away to college, I went as a "pretty girl," a piece of fluff with no sense of my former academic self-esteem. I wanted to get away from my home town, but I had lost most of my ambition to study. I was excited to meet lots of new guys. I was getting B's, some A's, a couple C's. Then I took a graduate-level course, called Classical Political Thought, with a female professor who affirmed my intellect. That experience changed my life.

In a private meeting, she told me that she and another professor had just had a conversation about me. "Your written work is brilliant, but for some reason you don't speak up in class or assert yourself. What's wrong?" She insisted that I had more potential than any student she had ever taught. It reawakened me to hear those words from someone for whom I had immense respect. It meant I was still smart, like I used to be! As an undergraduate, I got an A in that professor's class—one of only three A's in a class full of graduate students.

I started pouring my energy back into my studies to see if she was right, if I still had potential. It worked: I got A's and more A's. I became respected in my department as one of the political science hotshots. As a theorist and Marxian analyst, I have developed my own approach which has garnered compliments, and the more compliments I received for my work, the more motivated I became. I have also challenged myself to develop a "voice" in political science classes full of men.

In the past year or two, I have recognized that my ability is back. I am excited abut my future and my career: I want to be a university professor. Had my professor not observed my abilities, they would have stayed hidden. I would have pursued an "MRS" degree and would never have been able to mine all my potential. I am so indebted to her. That one comment was powerful enough to change my direction.

I have more confidence now, even when I go home and face lingering perceptions of me as a piece of meat or an intellectual lightweight. Unfortunately, in my extended family there is no place for a smart young woman; there is no place for a woman, period. Even though my sister is the smart one, she is not included in the men's debates. She is simply trotted out to provide a piece of trivia for the conversation; she is not allowed to engage in real discourse about the issues in which she has been formally educated. In our family circle, women occupy the servant role and everyone upholds that expectation.

At a recent family gathering, I was telling my 92-year-old grandfather about my upcoming trip to South Dakota to do research at an Indian reservation. The discussion soon turned into an argument with the other men about the Indian character. When I tried to discuss political and economic realities, I was summoned to the kitchen by my mom and the other women who said, "Don't start fighting with the guys!" As a woman in my family it has always been difficult to develop a "voice."

As a freshman in college, I was still doing myself up, wearing makeup and styling my hair every day. However, when I enrolled in a women's studies course, I began reading about how oppressive makeup and external image can be. I have become very aware of how media images encourage women to be beautiful, coy, gentle, fragile, and feminine. And insecure about their looks. In addition, they end up feeling bad about asserting themselves and unable to defend themselves. It's not nice!

Through that course, I began to see what I had done to myself because of images of femininity: wax my eyebrows, fill the gap between my teeth, agonize over food on a daily basis, hide my potential and my "voice"—all this torture in the name of beauty and popularity. When I came to that realization, I decided I wasn't going to do it anymore. I started to reclaim myself and gave up the image routines; it fit into my life perfectly because I was also undergoing a transformation in the academic arena. The two went together; I got away from the symbolism and developed my substance at the same time on a conscious level. I didn't want to be a toy any longer; I wanted to worry about the bigger issues.

Although I have worked on developing my "voice" and my assertiveness, I still have to force myself to speak up. When I do assert myself it always goes well, so I don't know why I'm still reluctant to do it. It's hard to get the words out of my mouth due to all those years of enforced passivity. It's a constant struggle to believe that my voice is worth hearing and that as a woman I matter.

Last Friday my roommate and I ordered carryout food but when the delivery man came my roommate was upstairs. I let him into the apartment because it was below freezing outside, but after I paid him he made no move to leave. He asked, "Who's here?" and didn't believe me when I said my roommate was upstairs. He started moving farther into the apartment to verify his assumption that I was alone, but when my roommate came clomping down the stairs, he ran out. Had I reacted the way I wanted to react, I would have screamed and cussed at him to leave. But at the risk of hurting someone's feelings, I did the nice thing.

As part of my upbringing, my mom always insisted that I not argue or question or be assertive. Make everyone happy. Smile. I resent it at times because I have had to take a lot of inappropriate behavior from other people in general, as well as in my personal relationships. I know I shouldn't take that kind of behavior and I will have to be much more assertive in graduate school, but I still don't want to "rock the boat." Perhaps if I had been trained to be assertive, I would more easily have kicked the delivery man out. Although I called the restaurant and complained about the man's behavior, they were only concerned about losing my business, not about how this man might treat other customers.

My college social life changed as my external and internal image changed. My first year in school, I primped, wore torturous fashions, and dated good-looking ultra-jocks. Now I prefer comfortable clothes and wear my hair naturally. As a result, I have attracted a different type of man. My boyfriend is a brilliant intellectual, on the fringes of society, with long hair and pierced ears, but this is the type of guy I want to attract. Had he met me my freshman year, he would never have been interested. When I changed myself, I changed the qualities I valued in other people as well.

Men—male friends and boyfriends—have always fed my self-image by telling me I'm attractive. They've been really supportive. My women friends have, too, but it's hard to have women friends who aren't jealous. I would love to believe that every woman is a sister, as women's studies teaches, but I've had a lot of bad experiences with women and jealousy. Women haven't been as supportive when I get insecure. I get backhanded compliments: "I hate you; you're so beautiful." I don't know how to take that. With women there's also my guilt over their bad feelings that I am more attractive. If we go out together, they're afraid that I'll meet all the men. It's so hard to make female friends. The other day a woman asked me if I knew how beautiful I was. My answer was, "sometimes."

Normally I am comfortable with my looks; sometimes I feel extraordinarily beautiful, and other times I feel downright ugly. I can make a direct correlation between how bad I feel about myself and how much TV I have watched. The fashion cable channel, for example, has very skinny fashion models interspersed with ads for the Sports Illustrated swimsuit edition and Playboy's Playmate of the Year edition, and ads for hair and diet products. I come away feeling that I have to lose weight, work out, start running. Of course, I know I can never look like those unreal women who have weight trainers, dieticians, hairdressers, makeup artists, and fashion designers putting them together. I know their photographs are airbrushed to remove any facial wrinkles or thigh bulges. Even Cindy Crawford looks like a normal woman—albeit with abnormally long legs—without all that help.

Women who are not able to pick apart these images and see the power relations, sexism, and exploitation can easily be influenced and made to feel insecure. Women's studies have helped me realize how much junk this is. For so long I bought the idea that my life could be better if my lips were redder and my lashes thicker. We are constantly striving for the better life portrayed by the women in the ads. I would love to see a real woman in an advertisement some day, and a significant realignment of what this culture thinks is beautiful.

When I think about myself as I am day to day, I feel really good about how far I've come. I have no desire to go back to the days when I was putting so much time and energy into the way I looked. I don't feel bad about wearing makeup; I still wear it once in a while, but now I'm aware of the reason that I wear it. I know it's oppressive, but I can choose to wear it or not. If you can't go out of the house without makeup because you feel horrible, that's one thing, but if you like wearing it and have some awareness of the reason, that's another.

Although today's society still does not recognize that women can be both intelligent and attractive, I believe I have grown into a well-rounded person who can be both attractive and smart. I think I look better than ever right now, even without makeup. In terms of my body image, I can now identify with pictures of Marilyn Monroe. By today's standards she was fuller-figured and, although by my standards she was thin, I think she looked like a woman, not a 14-year-old boy.

I think about the aging process all the time. My grandfather is 93 and still drives a car and tractor, chops wood, and goes to Florida. He is as mobile as anyone. So the idea of aging doesn't scare me. However, if I end up immobilized I will be absolutely miserable. I want to make a conscientious effort to stay active. I have started thinking about current lifestyle factors that may affect my future health.

As far as looks are concerned, there is a huge bias against older women—"Women grow older, men grow dignified." That bothers me in theory, but I hope to figure out how to deal with it as I grow older. People make fun of the gray-haired older-woman image, but it's also endearing. I can identify with the grandmotherly type, but I'd also like to be feisty. I don't want to be stagnant. It's really what you make of it. I'll just have to see how it goes.

JOAN, 55
psychotherapist

As a young child, I remember sitting on the couch in the living room with my feet just barely extended over the edge. For the rest of my life I have been tall, so it's quite pleasant to remember the sensation of being little. I also remember being thrown back and forth between my father and my uncle; that's how I learned to like things that were scary. I realized there was some danger, but it was so much fun flying through the air between the two of them.

Later I remember feeling tall, but until puberty it was not a concern. I was always just taller; even in kindergarten and first grade I was always in the back row of the group pictures. Always as tall as the boys and sometimes taller, at age 12 I was 5'9", 148 pounds, and really built.

I think I was fairly obnoxious as a kid—a spoiled only child and happily so, the center of my parents' attention. For as long as I can remember I had a very clear picture of the kind of person I wanted to be, which included being straightforward and honest. My parents raised me to tell the truth by not punishing me if I did. Whether or not others had a problem with my forthrightness, it was what my parents expected of me. Later in life I came to realize I had been a leader in almost every group I had been in because I was willing to state what I wanted. I was rewarded for behavior that could be considered selfish or spoiled.

I was pretty secure in the things I had learned in my family, and that included being demonstrative. Both my parents were affectionate and we'd hug and kiss in public, but I remember seeing disapproving or uncomfortable responses from other people.

I grew up as an affectionate child who kissed family and friends upon meeting. It was a way of exploring: feeling, smelling, and kissing cheeks. My mother always asked me what I did on dates, and it occurred to me later that it wasn't just motherly concern but curiosity. She managed to hug and kiss any boy I dated. She liked feeling the guys. I like feeling them and I like the smell of them, too. So I am my mother's daughter in those sensuous ways, while my father talked about ideas and taught me to think prior to decisions and actions.

Dad and I talked about all kinds of stuff; he shared more and revealed more of himself. My mother was more self-contained and less interesting but, at the same time, comfortable to be around and easy to talk to. And a good hugger. I used to think that I learned hugging at my father's knee, but when I got older I realized that my mother was the one who would melt right into a hug. My father was more uptight. I am sure he was more comfortable with me physically when I was younger, but even then he was always more uptight than my mother. He and I were unusually close, however. He actually said that he told me more things and was more vulnerable with me than with any other person in his life.

When my body changed at age 12 1/2, I was really pleased with how I looked—but that was the only year I enjoyed it. Although I didn't get a bra until I realized that walking down the stairway in school caused me to bounce and be uncomfortable, I started off with a 34B. At that point everything about my body was just about right. Except for my nose.

From age 13 I had been unhappy with my nose and wanted to have it fixed. At that age my mother said I was too young for plastic surgery, but if I was still unhappy at 18 we would talk about it. I had a Roman nose with a bump on the bridge and a little point on the end. It looked okay from the front, but I was so self-conscious about my profile that if I couldn't sit in the back of the bus, I would sit facing the back to avoid being seen from the side. By the time I was halfway through my first year of college, however, I had decided that I had adjusted to my nose. Then my mother said I was old enough to have the operation, and a school friend encouraged me because she had had hers done. I had the surgery at the end of my freshman year in college. Afterwards my dad commented, "Joanie, I liked your old nose but it required a dignity that someone your age has trouble carrying off. Now your expressions fit your face." My nose still has most of its character, but I'm not self-conscious about my profile any more.

I was also self-conscious about my long feet and frustrated with the meager selection of decent shoes. In high school I wouldn't be caught dead in the ever-popular saddle shoes because my feet looked even bigger. So I lived in suede loafers and big, thick Wigwam socks, which I cuffed to help minimize the size of my feet. Because my mother always made sure my shoes fit properly, my feet were never scrunched, but I am beginning to run out of room in my size 12s now. In size 13 there will be no selection whatsoever!

As a kid I was normal to skinny. The first time I gained weight was at age 15, working as a soda jerk and savoring ice cream every day. I gained 15 pounds and then stayed the same weight for years until I went to graduate school, where I picked up another 25 pounds out of anxiety. But even inside my currently heavy body there is a shapely, attractive young woman.

I am built very much like my mother, who was always very attractive in a natural way. Both my parents thought I was a good-looking kid and I thought they were nifty parents. All my friends loved to come over and visit. My mother sat in on my parties, and when we had kissing games she participated! She was very popular. There was never any sense of competition; we admired each other. Because she looked younger and I looked older, people always asked if we were sisters.

As a freshman in high school, I looked older, was more mature, and wore sweaters that were too tight; I was just more than most guys that age could handle. I didn't know if comments like "Big Mother!" from the boys were intended to hurt or insult me. By the end of the year, disliking all the sexual attention I was getting, I realized it was not safe to look so sexy.

So I cut my hair and wore nothing but blouses for the next two years in hopes of projecting a more asexual image. I didn't really like the way I looked, but I wasn't pestered so much. I had liked feeling like a sexually attractive female, but those comments made me feel put down by guys I sometimes didn't even know. So when I ran into one of those ill-spoken fellows again at the neighborhood YMCA, I went over to him and said, "If you ever speak to me that way again, I'll slap your face!" I felt self-respecting enough to stand up for myself; I didn't just take it.

I never considered myself popular in high school. I was friendly with everybody, but I didn't date much. I don't remember boys asking me out.

After college I worked as a secretary at a mental health clinic for about four years before realizing I wanted to do psychotherapy. During that time I met some social work students who came for supervision while they "practiced" psychotherapy at our clinic. At age 25 I was becoming interested in graduate school, so I asked those students what was involved. The master's degree in social work was a two-year program with a group project, which sounded easier than writing a thesis. Also, I understood a Ph.D. in psychology would have taken seven years, and a psychiatric medical degree was out of the question. So social work was my most direct route to becoming a psychotherapist. Once I decided I wanted to go to graduate school, I applied to and was accepted at the University of Chicago.

Over the years, I have attended a number of grammar school and high school reunions, which provided some very interesting personal feedback. I had had no idea of the impression I made on people; I thought I was friendly, had fun in class, liked most of the other kids, and was fairly dependable.

However, at these reunions I learned that I had been considered destined to be different. At one of my grammar school gatherings, the women's exclusive profile was: marriage and children, a typical life for people of my generation. And there I was with a master's degree in social work and my own private practice, a first marriage at age 45 to a man 16 years my junior, and no children. My classmates were not at all surprised, saying, "We always knew you were going be different." I didn't know why they had seen that; my own perception was simply that I had had more sense of self.

From some of the men at those reunions, I discovered an even more interesting concept: several of them had seen me as someone to fantasize about. In those years I was hiding my hurt feelings regarding boys by acting aloof and sophisticated as protection from the social scene. At the time it hadn't occurred to me that I might have been intimidating to those same boys. Their comments put things into perspective for me.

In my senior year of college I made friends with a woman who is still my closest friend and who, apart from my parents, had the most impact on my becoming the person I wanted to be. As a role model for me, she clearly had a set of values that were difficult to attain and by which she tried to live. She was also very good at intellectual discussion and argument. She defined for me what friendship entailed, and ultimately we forged a really good relationship because we were both very clear about what we wanted: commitment and appropriate behavioral values. She has always been the person I look to for feedback, problem solving, and direction. When I would get off the track, she would help me clarify my values and keep me close to my own agenda. And I provided her with comfort, playfulness, and the warmth she needed. I got her comfortable with hugging. She has continued to influence the way I am and the way I perceive myself.

When I finally met my future husband, I told him that my women friends give me things no man can give and they will always have an important place in my life. He said, "Okay!" It tickles me that he's such a feminist. He really likes women. Somehow I had had a terrible picture of what a husband was like. In my mind the nicest, most eligible guy would turn into the worst chauvinist pig the minute he became a husband.

There were two other major self-image boosting experiences in my life. In my 30s I worked with a woman therapist who had a lot of charisma, a quality I have always envied but also mistrusted. This woman had an impressive intensity, engaging others with a laser-like manner that I always found uncomfortable and intimidating. Through my dealings with her, I was finally able to clarify in my own mind the difference between intensity and depth: a person can have strong personal feelings but not necessarily understand someone else's feelings. And the feedback I was getting from others was that I had depth of understanding, empathy, and appreciation for people, whether or not I had intensity. I can't tell you how moving that discovery was for me!

The other incident involves a visit to an adult education school in northern Wisconsin. One of the classes was given by a wonderful teacher, a Ph.D. in political science. There were, among twenty-five students in the class, three women: a writer who had known him for a long time, a very bright friend of mine, and me. It turned out that we were the stars who kept the class discussions going. Although I didn't really think I was stupid, I hadn't had a real sense of my smarts until then. In planning a skit for the three of us to present, I made suggestions that the other two members of my triad thought were great. So in that same week I also discovered I was creative.

Over the years there have also been many other experiences that improved my self-image by improving my self-confidence. Most taught me to stand up for my rights and defend myself verbally. This increased verbal assertiveness combined with my impressive physical presence has given me a real sense of my own power.

Using tough language was something I discovered early—at the age of 14 or 15. I was in a sorority in high school and we had baseball games all over a large area of empty lots in Hyde Park. In the middle of one of these games, a kid who was maybe a year younger—this little short kid—came along and took our bat! I felt responsible because I was the president of the sorority. So I said, "Give us back our bat, we're in the middle of a game!" His response was, "Come and get it!" So I ran after him, but I couldn't catch him. Finally, I was so frustrated I stopped and just yelled out every swear word I had ever learned at school—not at home, my parents never swore. He stopped, turned around, looked at me as if to say, "Ugh!" and dropped the bat with great emphasis on how terrible I was for using such language. And I thought, "Gee, using your mouth works! None of this chasing people. This is what works." That was a real lesson and I occasionally found it to be most effective.

Years later as a therapist-in-training, I participated in a required and long-term assignment which consisted of going out alone in order to learn how to meet people on my own. I actually learned a great deal from this experience. I didn't stay alone for long and people were still interested in me even if I wore my glasses. (I never used to wear them, but I couldn't see the person I was responding to, until he got up close and then I wasn't always interested.) What I hadn't yet learned was how to keep people I didn't want in my apartment, out of my apartment. In any case, I had picked up a guy in the bar in the Playboy Towers which was my usual haunt for this exercise. We had gone out for dinner and he had come back to my apartment. But by then he was coming on to me and I said, "I'm sorry, but I'm not interested." We were standing in my living room and he became really pissed. So I finally said, "Listen, if you figured you would buy me dinner and get a free fuck, I'll give you your money back!" Standing eye to eye and nose to nose with him, I literally saw him think about hitting me. But then he thought better of it. I really used my height and verbal skills to deal with him.

Six or seven years ago, two friends and I went to Madison to attend the Drum Corp International competition. Unfortunately, we came in the wrong end of the stadium almost at starting time. With my friends ahead of me, we began to make our way down the whole length of the stadium, just as the band started to play the Canadian national anthem. Everyone was standing still, but we were moving along toward our seats. Suddenly, this 50-something guy about my height who was balding, grey-haired, and bulbous-nosed said, "Oh no, you are not getting past me!" He was very disapproving. Now, I agreed that we should have been giving proper respect to the Canadian national anthem, however, somehow it just pissed me off! So I said, "Get out of here!" I got right up to the guy, and I mean in his face! I said to him, "You can do what you want to do, but you don't tell me what to do!" He replied with, "You bitch, I ought to slap you!" And I said, leaning forward even closer, "You would!" He backed off. And we moved! I have come to appreciate more and more my height. I've learned it's harder for people to depreciate or patronize me if I'm looking at them eye to eye. There was something about being physical in that way. There was no danger. He wasn't going to slug me in that crowd of people. But being intimidating—moving into his space—was just thrilling because as a female I don't often get to do that.

And then one time right here in the neighborhood, at Wrightwood and Lakeview, I encountered a car that was trying to insinuate itself into the line of traffic. The person ahead of me denied the driver access and so did I. Finally he got into line behind me. When I got to the stop sign at the four-way intersection there was a car to my right signaling to make a left turn in front of me. Recognizing that car's right-of-way, I didn't move but the car behind me honked. I got pissed! I'm quick to emotion and that's one of the emotions I'm quick to. Then he really got annoyed at my delay and as I made my right turn he turned with me—into the oncoming traffic lane, except there were no cars coming on Lakeview. When he rolled his window down, I rolled mine down. And he said, "What's the idea?" Now, I was not necessarily lucid in that state so I said, "Fuck you!" He responded with, "What kind of way is that for a lady to talk?" And I said, "I don't give a shit what you think of me!" He finally moved on, but he stayed in the wrong lane as he went because there were so many cars in line ahead of me in my lane. No one let him into our lane, and traffic began to pile up in front of him in his lane, with him going in the wrong direction. So when I got up to him I gave him the obscene gesture and just kept going. He turned off as soon as he could. Finally, it occurred to me that this behavior just wasn't smart and I should have been more careful, because he might have been one of those guys with a gun in his glove compartment. It was fun at the moment but I haven't done anything that gross since then!

Through these experiences, I have learned to use my hard-won physicality and verbal abilities effectively. At this point in my life, I know that I can handle myself successfully in any situation that comes along. It's a great feeling!

As I've gotten older, I've become more like my mother who enjoyed telling people what she thought and who felt freer to do so as she got older. I've gotten into the habit of telling people all kinds of things that I'm thinking just because I can do it now. I give people compliments all the time, but only when I mean it.

The most fun incident happened recently when I spent an evening volunteering and saw the best-looking guy there. He was probably in his late 20s or early 30s. He wasn't the type I normally go for, but I liked his looks. So at the end of the evening I went over and sat next to him and said, "I just wanted to tell you that I have enjoyed looking at you all night!" He was really pleased. And I told him that at this age I say what I think. "I like the bone structure, the features, the shoulders—the whole thing looks nice."

He said, "Thank you very much, but why did you preface your remarks with 'at this age?'" I explained that if I had made that comment at a younger age the person might read more into it than I had intended. They would assume it was some kind of come-on. And then I'd have to deal with that. But at this age it's less likely to take that turn. Then he said, "I think that's too bad!" I assured him that usually people are only interested in other people their own age or younger. And he said, "Well, I think that's a waste!" So I said obviously my husband does too because he's sixteen years younger, so thank you very much! It was as if we had a thing for each other. And as it turned out, we later ran into each other in the lobby of my building where he had been living for several months. He was sitting in the lobby and we looked at each other as I was walking out. He did a double-take and I said, "It's you!" We almost hugged. It was really funny! And of course I had no intentions of doing anything other than just enjoying his person. That was fun.

I used to like certain looks on a woman: dark hair and eyes, exotic features. At a party once I spotted a younger woman I thought was very attractive and then she came over to me and said, "Don't you think we look a lot alike?" That was neat. But should I be embarrassed for admiring people who look similar to me?

Now that I am older, my looks often depend on the light or the angle at which I am seen. Sometimes I look young and sexy and sometimes I just look middle-aged and overweight. But at some point I stopped agonizing about losing weight; I don't care as much anymore. My husband's happy with me. For health reasons it would be fine to lose weight, so I try not to gain, but I am not willing to agonize over being less than perfect. Part of me would like to look great in anything, but I can afford better clothes these days, so I can rely on clothes more and on my body less. Unless your weight is harmful to your health, how you look is such a superficial concern. I am really tired of it, and yo-yo dieting is the worst.

The first time I had the shock of seeing myself on film was postgraduate school, at age 31, when I was overweight, wearing inexpensive clothes, and going without makeup except for lipstick. Although I didn't see myself as particularly attractive or sexual, I did see someone who fit my idea of an intellectual New York Jew—the whole stereotype. But I also saw that I was not attending to being female or sexual; I was all head and I really didn't like what I saw! So, although I had been openly resistant to the traditional female image with cosmetic jars and bottles, I went for a makeup lesson. There, for the first time, I discovered the magic of blusher. What a change! As soon as I started wearing blusher, people asked about my new eye makeup or my contact lenses! They knew something was different and thought it must be my eyes.

I didn't see myself on tape again for many years until my husband and I appeared on a television program about nontraditional marriages. We were "the older woman and younger man." That was interesting from a different perspective. I was 46, and looking more middle-aged with some excess weight. I didn't look as good as I would have liked, but when I talked, my face was so expressive! I liked that very much. I had never seen myself that way; I was not animated on the first tape at age 31.

When Jimmy and I were planning to get married and I pointedly told people about our age difference, nine out of ten people rushed to reassure me, "It doesn't matter. What matters is that you love each other." That cracked me up every time: I wasn't asking for reassurance—I was bragging that I had bagged a young one! Their reassurance was certainly not what I expected.

I am very happy with my life. I have done things that for many people are just fantasies, things to dream about or read about in a book. There is always room for improvement but I now think of myself as a strong person, comfortable and effective. I used to get angry, throw tantrums, and be totally ineffectual. And I was always such a chicken. I had to work for years to develop guts, to be more spontaneous and outgoing, and to stay out of my head. Every now and then I would do something risky and find it wasn't that hard, but the hard things were big accomplishments that I really had to work at. And, because many of the things I have always done were easy, I didn't credit myself with them, although they impressed other people. In that area and in some small way I can compare myself with my upstairs neighbor, an amazingly wonderful artist, who has always been creative so he doesn't think much of it.

JOANI, 45:
human resources consultant

My first memory of myself was my image in a mirror, all dressed in pink—a lot of pink! I didn't think pink was good on me, and it was not my favorite crayon color, either. This dress had ruffles and fancy attachments, bows and frilly froufrou nonsense. It was a special present from my grandma for my third birthday. Even as a young child, I knew that dress was not right for the real me. At the time I couldn't put it into words, but I realized I was dressed in something that someone else had selected. I came to understand much later that I had always worn things that fit somebody else's idea of who I was, rather than who I thought I was.

Looking back, that first memory was both a positive and negative experience: negative because I didn't like the dress or the way I looked in it; positive because I realized I was entitled to my own opinion. And in my family that was not easy to come by.

I grew very rapidly and very early. I was 5' 10", my adult height, by the time I was 12 years old. Every summer was one big incredible growth spurt from age 5 to age 12. I desperately wanted to fit in with the other kids, who were all six to ten inches shorter than I was.

Particularly around boys, I wanted to appear as short as possible—hence my posture was going to hell. My mother initiated posture lessons and eight years of very disciplined ballet for me. She felt that my sister and I had to learn to be proud of our height. Although my sister is 6', she grew at a much slower rate and continued growing until she was 18 or 19 years old, so she had a much easier time acclimating herself to her height. I was constantly surprised, constantly annoyed, and constantly trying to compensate.

In grade school, I was taller than the principal, all my teachers, and all the students. It wasn't until junior year in high school that a few of the boys and some of the male teachers were taller than I was. In my grade school pictures, with everyone lined up by height, I am always the first person in the back row.

A simple thing like shopping for shoes and winter coats was impossible. We'd shop in August when the coats first arrived in the stores, and yet find only one or two in my size that could be lengthened. In the miniskirt days, when coats couldn't be lengthened much, I had to have my coats made. A friend's invitation to go shopping, which was intended as an afternoon's adventure, was always humiliating, embarrassing, and unfruitful for me. There was a very limited selection of clothes because things in my size were for women, not young girls. So the colors, the styles, and the fabrics were always wrong but they were the only things available. On the bright side, the one thing I could count on was growing some more, so I wore most of those clothes for only one season!

The biggest issue was that I was very uncoordinated and gawky. I was always either falling down or walking into something. I was constantly bruised as a kid and constantly in the school nurse's office bleeding from an injury. So I came to see my body as the enemy. It would never cooperate with me. And just when I got used to the current phase, another growth spurt would hit and I'd be into a new phase.

I felt extremely ugly as a kid. I had gotten glasses at a young age. From 12 to 16 I was thin and gawky. My hair was extremely straight and wouldn't "bubble" in the current style. Everything about me was wrong. My father wouldn't let us wear makeup, so we'd sneak into the girls' bathroom at school and apply black eyeliner and white lipstick. Really flattering!

Because I was awkward and growing by leaps and bounds, I knew I had to compensate with my personality, to draw attention to myself but away from my body. The easiest way for me to do that was with my mouth. I come from a long line of talkers, big loud talkers. And I have been gifted with a terrific vocabulary. I learned that to be funny, witty, and quick with my mouth was the easiest way to draw attention away from my body, the bad clothes, the bad colors, and the look that wasn't me. Where I grew up, verbal skill was also a way to gain respect.

To say that my parents sent mixed messages about self-esteem is an understatement. On one hand, you could be anything you wanted if you studied and worked hard enough. On the other hand, you had to be exactly what they wanted you to be or you would be denied their approval, which in our house was the gift of love. Food was another gift of love. Both my parents had grown up during the Depression and were determined to give their children the best of everything. We benefited from exposure to lots of wonderful things, but we were also exposed to a lot of food we didn't need. And when I didn't get my parents' approval, I drowned that little girl inside me with food. That was, and still is, a negative experience in my life.

In our house, the game was that when we met certain standards, the standards were raised. Finally, when I was 15 years old, getting straight A's, working a part-time job, and enjoying tons of friends, I realized that my parents still didn't think I was good enough. So I gave up. I just decided that I needed to find my own way. I got approval from my friends and teachers, so I spent a lot of time out of the house. And to this day, if I want assurance about who I am, I never go to family—I always go to friends.

My friends and I were all devout subscribers to *Seventeen* magazine, our bible. And by seventh grade I had learned to use Simplicity patterns to do some very simple sewing. My art teacher suggested that I put together a fashion show for the rest of the student body. So I pulled out all my Simplicity patterns and put together what *Seventeen* magazine said was hot for spring. I made all the clothes and some of my friends modeled. It was a huge success! And I really, really liked doing it. That teacher had the most amazing effect on my self-image. She showed me that making decisions for myself about fashion was a way to please people and also please myself. It was another small but successful attempt to make decisions for myself. That was a big lesson, because in my house independent thinking was just not allowed.

Other influential people in my life were my friend Judy and her mother. Judy was the only girl in a family of four boys. Her mother doted on her like a little doll: new dresses for every day of the week, and all the hairpieces, jewelry, purses, and shoes to complete the ensemble. Her closet was like a store. I'd go over to her house after school and watch her mom put together the next day's outfit! I learned about color and pattern mixing, and trying new combinations. Experiment! Lay a sweater on the bed and throw different things at it and see how it worked. It was wonderful to see someone have fun with clothes. For me clothes were never fun; they were always an ordeal, a punishment. Clothes always said that I was the wrong size, the wrong weight, the wrong height, the wrong everything. Even when I looked pulled together or attractive, it always felt bad.

At some point in high school, even with my newly acquired contact lenses, I realized that I was never going to look like anybody else. I had started gaining weight quickly at age 17. I was extremely tall and my personality had become very outgoing. My clothes and my looks were never going to fit in. What finally reassured me about myself was the change in the dress code at school at the end of my junior year. We finally got to wear blue jeans to school. That was great. Now I could buy boys' clothes that looked just like girls' clothes. I could really look like everybody else, forget about the image I was projecting through clothing, and just worry about my grades.

In college, of course, in the middle of the Vietnam War, blue jeans were the standard uniform. Blue jeans, BVD T-shirts in a hundred colors, long underwear for the winter, and some sweaters. I was absolutely happy. I never worried about what I wore, because everybody wore the same thing. And it felt good. In those days, blue jeans had embroidery all over them, and because my grandmothers had taught me to crotchet, knit, and do tatting, I became very successful at decorating all my friends' jeans for them. So suddenly I was "in" when it came to clothing expertise in a pretty silly fashion world.

College was a real pleasure, a freeing experience. I could finally determine my look and my personality; nobody said "No!" I could now indulge all my creative urges, which had been stifled by others' expectations of me and by a lack of my own decision-making power. And there were so many people to meet. If one person didn't like me, there were ten others who liked the person I had become. So the years between 18 and 24 were really, really strong years for me.

Once in the working world, I had to constantly adjust my wardrobe for various full-time and part-time jobs. Teaching school at night, I wore things left from college. During the day I worked in a boutique and had to wear the latest styles. I was now enslaved to *Vogue* magazine, but it still wasn't appropriate for me. Later, in the corporate world, there were all the dress codes: little bow ties and those awful navy suits. Because everyone wore the uniform, it was easy to fit in, but again I was dressing to please someone else. And my body was still the enemy. I had put on a lot of weight in college. My hatred of my height and weight was intensified by wearing corporate clothes that didn't work with my body.

When I had been in the corporate environment about eight years, my mom saw an ad in the paper for a boutique for sizes 2-20, petite through tall! Could this be true? I called. The owner, Alice, was 6' herself. I had finally found a woman who was taller than I and who was actually interested in clothing. She proposed to make me look like the real me. And for the next five years, while I spent nearly every dime on clothes, she was pretty successful. Alice truly understood "tall" as well as elegance and classic style. I still could not carry off gracefulness, but I was elegantly dressed at last.

During that time, I also went through a lot of therapy to get at the root of all my weight changes and the reason I was using food disadvantageously. So, while I was still under Alice's fashion tutelage, I lost more than eighty pounds. The fashions that she created for me and the way she helped me define my personal style were wonderful gifts. She taught me how to compensate for my height and weight with a certain presence. Gradually, she helped me give up the chronic worry of how to dress, what to wear, and how to fit in.

While working in a very conservative bank, I woke up every morning knowing I was the best-dressed person in the place. I knew that when I gave a speech or conducted a seminar, everybody's eyes would be on me for the right reasons. When I got compliments on those clothes, I knew people weren't being charitable; they were as impressed as I was. And so for the first time, my height, weight, and coloring—the real me—was packaged perfectly. That was such a euphoric feeling; it can never be duplicated. Unfortunately, Alice closed her store and I was just devastated! Although I could still spend time with someone who truly understood what it was like to be tall, I could no longer buy her product.

Over the years, I've learned that my appearance has less to do with who I am and, certainly, less to do with how people care about me than I originally thought. I now understand that appearance is a variable that can be used to help me, to draw people to me, as well as to keep people away from me—something in my bag of tricks, to use at will. I have learned to use clothes as a powerful tool, so my clothes are congruent with my physical appearance and what I am really saying about myself.

At my age, I don't have to look at the fashion magazines anymore and say, "This is who I have to be this season." I know I can wear the classic, elegant styles Alice created for me; I don't have to worry about what everybody else is wearing. The conclusion I came to in high school is definitely true: I am never going to be like anybody else. But frankly, now that I am more secure about who I am, I am glad I'm unique.

The first descriptive word I would choose for my physical self is obviously fat. I am enormously overweight right now and I need to lose weight. But a better term, which other people have used, is "overwhelming." When people first meet me, they are bowled over. My package is large, tall, loud, and dressed in bright colors. It can be a "whelming" experience to be confronted by me!

But the other words that I use to describe myself are negative, because I still don't have a very positive image. I think about myself positively only in the future tense. Some day I am going to be the elegant, thin person of my imagination; it's always just beyond my grasp.

The face I expose to the outside world is a much more positive face than the one I see in the mirror. I am enormously critical of myself, although I have pretty exacting standards for everybody else as well. Right now my face and my body are congruent with who I am. I have just started my own business, so the rules are mine to make. There is no dress code— no more "ladylike" look of Mother's, no more professional "knock 'em dead with my intellect" image that my father insisted on, and surely no more *Seventeen* or *Vogue*. I really have come into my own. I get to choose my clothes and my colors. My face and body, although certainly not my ideal proportion, fit my personality. I have a large personality and a large frame that seem to go together these days. The colors I wear are symbolic of the things I like about myself. These bright, open, and forthright colors are appealing to me and they represent how I project myself.

Unfortunately, I don't see myself as positively as others see me. Most people attribute far too much to me. I don't really think I possess all those qualities. The day I am at peace with myself is the day I have as positive an image of myself as my friends have. Most people compliment me on being very warm, giving, funny, intelligent, and vivacious. If I compliment myself on anything, it's on being a good friend. Often when I am tired and don't feel like the belle of the ball, I do it anyway because I've got this image to live up to that I have created.

Although I am happier with myself than I have ever been, I am not totally happy with me. I really need to learn to give myself a break. I am so hard on myself. I will never be smart enough, quick enough, pretty enough, nice enough, caring enough, intellectual enough. I strive to improve constantly because Joani just isn't good enough. And that truly is a family message.

Dealing with the aging process? I buy a lot of Clinique! I really spend money on that stuff—I take very good care of my skin, which is very good in its own right and a legacy of our family. I eat good things, a balanced diet, even if it's way too much. My hair is a goner. It's thinning out fast. Because of my excessive weight, I worry about diseases associated with aging: osteoporosis, diabetes, and, certainly, heart disease. If I worry about the aging process at all, I worry about it in terms of physical health.

When I think about the future, I know exactly what I'm going to look like. All my female relatives lived to a very old age, so I'm familiar with the face. I am not going to tamper with plastic surgery. I want my face to look as if I have had a very interesting life.

If there is one thing women can help other women with, particularly younger women, it's solid advice about clothes as only one part of the person you become. Unfortunately in our society, too much emphasis is placed on the packaging, not the contents of the package. Women spend their whole youth slaving after an ideal they can't achieve. It would be helpful if women received information to help them look really good for who they are—not for who's on the cover of *Vogue* magazine, but for their shape, their personality, and their lifestyle. This would surely help.

Also, we need to be more charitable toward other women. We come in all shapes and sizes and colors, and it's about time we started respecting each other for the way we are, not the way we are expected to be. I see lots of middle-aged women having plastic surgery and liposuction because they still don't have any confidence in who they are. They want to be what the latest magazine cover says they should be. Women are the only ones who can help other women put a stop to that.

JOANNE, 37:
sales

My first memory of my appearance as a child is of being dressed exactly like my sister, as if we were twins. Although there are two years between us, we were dressed identically on Christmas and other holidays. We even got the same dolls and gifts from my mother and dad.

As we got older, my sister and I became total opposites. She got up two hours before school, did her hair and makeup, and put on a dress and heels. I got up minutes before school, threw on my blue jeans and a T-shirt, and took off. We fought a lot. I didn't want to be like her, so I did the opposite of what she did all through high school and into our 20s.

My father managed to make both my sister and me feel that we were his favorite. He pulled a good trick on us in that way. I feel I was his real favorite; I was Daddy's little girl. When we played cards at grandpa's house, my father always sat by me. If I got the Old Maid, he would take it from me so I wouldn't get stuck with it! He always protected me.

My sister has always been my mother's favorite child. They are a lot alike; they even look alike. Then too, my sister has followed "The Plan According to Mother," whereas I'm probably a disappointment to her. She can't control me and she expected something different from me. Naturally, I like to think I look like my dad and take after his side of the family.

My father was tall and good-looking as a young man. My mother was 18 when she married him. He wasn't much of a provider: The small settlement he received from the driver who disabled him in an automobile accident was completely spent after six years of drinking. After having five children, my mother divorced him, perhaps thinking she could do better.

My parents divorced in 1963 when I was 8. I can remember the day my father left. I went into their bedroom where he was putting his things into a cardboard box on the bed. When I asked where he was going, he told me he had to go away for a while. And that's the last time he stayed with us. I don't really know why my mother divorced my father, nor do I know why she remarried.

I was the youngest of five until I was 11 years old. By then my mother had remarried and my half-brother was born. Mother's second husband was also alcoholic as well as verbally abusive. My sister and I became very close in those years, clinging to each other in bed when the arguments, threats of abandonment, and yelling got loud and scary. Mother said the reason she stayed in the second marriage was that she could not face another divorce and the responsibility of raising six children alone.

Because of Mother's remarriage there was the additional trauma of moving from Wisconsin to Kentucky—a very alien environment—when I was in fifth grade. My stepfather was much better off financially than my father had been, so we began moving in an upper-middle-class social circle. It was nice but it was also anxiety provoking. We had to do things just so, and be just so, which only exacerbated my existing feelings of insecurity. I had no sense of identity in grade school and high school and this part of my young life filled me with fear, dread, and anxiety that still permeate my life and self-image. I think the family situation and moving to a new place had greatly undermined any confidence I might have had in myself.

However, one of the good things about living in that small southern town was that my parents belonged to the country club and we had to learn the social graces of meeting people and conversing. Mother was always big on the social stuff and I always balked. Most of our fights were over the way I dressed. Throughout high school and college, I wasn't the least bit fashion conscious. I seldom dressed up; I wore the standard uniform of jeans and T-shirts. My mother's standard line was, "You are not leaving the house looking like that. What if somebody sees you?" Of course I didn't care what anyone thought because my mother cared so tremendously. To make matters worse, my stepfather worked in one of the best companies in town at that time and had a position to uphold in the community. I was considered a reflection on both my mother and him, and I wasn't holding up my end of the deal.

The first time I walked into my new classroom in Kentucky, I overheard someone say, "Oh, she's kind of cute but kind of fat." I still remember the dress I had on: It was empire waisted, in royal blue with green embroidery, and a thin grosgrain ribbon that tied and hung down in the front. I had loved that dress and was so proud of the way I looked, but I don't think I ever wore it again after that dreadful day.

Between the ages of 5 and 14, I was overweight, probably because of the family situation, the divorce, remarriage, and the move. The summer before high school I lost 30 pounds; when I started school, people who had known me in eighth grade didn't recognize me. However, as a freshman I was still the typical ugly duckling: I wasn't fat anymore but I still had braces and glasses. I was fairly intelligent but I wasn't popular. I never had a boyfriend; I wasn't a cheerleader. As a result, I fell into the druggie-hippie group.

We were a middle-class, fairly well-off group of kids. Though our parents made more money than the average parents in our high school, we came to school in jeans and T-shirts and smoked pot. We had more fun going out with our girls' group on Friday and Saturday nights than we did with boyfriends. I really wasn't that interested in boys. Maybe that was my reaction to not being sought after, or maybe I was just covering up because a lot of my friends had boyfriends. They started kissing boys in the fifth grade and wearing their little basketball charms on a chain. They made dates to meet at the roller rink or the movies. The peer pressure was awful. I hated it!

As I got older I got cuter, so by the time I was a senior I was pretty cute. But I still wasn't very interested in boys. One boy asked me out, but when I found out how dumb he was, I lost interest. Cute-but-stupid wasn't for me. As a high school senior I went to a James Taylor concert and finally met somebody there whom I thought was pretty smart. He was a year older and in college. He was the first boy I dated and it lasted for about four years.

Our high school didn't have much in the line of women's sports' programs, so I hardly ever participated in sports. I was always the last person picked for all the team sports, especially baseball. They made us play all the things I wasn't good at. Other things like swimming or running or cross-country skiing were never offered. So because I wasn't good at team sports, there was nothing else to balance my life with and nothing else to build on.

When I got into college, I didn't have a lot of free time; I had to maintain my grades to keep my scholarship. I was busy all the time with classes, studying and working. I really liked my job in the graduate school records office and began to feel a sense of belonging. I was doing well academically and enjoying friendships and activities.

My senior year of college was difficult, however. I broke up with the guy I had met at the concert. All my friends were his friends, so when we broke up he kept all the friends and I had none. I started running to make myself feel better. The exercise was good but I was still all by myself, living alone for the first time because my roommate had gotten married. It was awfully depressing. When I got out of college I felt emotionally weak.

Initially I went home to my family. Then I realized I had to make a fast break, otherwise I might never get out of there. So I moved to Chicago, which was both brave and foolish because I really wasn't prepared for it. I found a job and an apartment downtown. Those two and a half years I lived alone in that tiny apartment in Chicago were the most frightening years of my life. The loneliness and the responsibility for my own welfare were overwhelming.

My first year in Chicago was 1977-78, and it was a terrible winter! We had never had weather like that in Kentucky, so I had no winter coat or boots. I had no money and my parents didn't give me any. I think they forgot about me. I surely could have used a little more support from them at that point in my life.

I have been embarrassed and saddened that I had never gotten to know my father better because he was an interesting person. So, when I moved to Chicago I saw him on a fairly regular basis for two or three years, but he passed away when I was only 28. What effect he had on me I don't know. I feel that he was truly proud of my accomplishments. He wanted me to go to school and marry well but he wanted me to do it for myself.

My mother wanted me to go to school so I wouldn't get trampled on or be too dependent. Her attitude was so defensive. My mother's admonitions to be independent, get an education, take care of myself, avoid dependence on men have taken root, however. I feel compelled to make money and prove myself over and over again in my career.

In business situations I feel comfortable, but I am uncomfortable and insecure at parties or in large groups. Anything over six people and I feel I have nothing to contribute. What could anybody possibly find interesting in me? I have accepted myself to the point of not going to large parties because I don't enjoy them; I won't put myself through that any more.

In business, however, I handle myself very well—so well that it even surprises me. I also know I've accomplished a lot, but it's not enough. I thought that by my late 30s I would be a famous writer, or would have contributed something to the world. But I haven't done anything. I am having a lot of anxiety about what I am doing, where I am going, and how my past has shaped me.

I can say all is not yet lost; I am only going to be 38 in February. But time passes so quickly. I felt the best about myself when I was in my early 30s. I was in good physical shape and had a very responsible job. I definitely felt I was at the top at that point in my life. Yet I've had only two career-type jobs in my life, which shows I'm not much of a risk taker. I feel the need to get a new job to prove that I can climb the corporate ladder again.

When I got my MBA, I thought I could lay back and relax in my career. I have closed myself off from other opportunities in my job for the past seven years. At this point I feel I've wasted at least three years by coasting in what is now a dead-end job. And I don't want to be caught off-guard like that again. Or maybe I'm being too hard on myself. I have done a lot but it's hard for me to admit it.

Interestingly enough, I have often thought that my appearance was responsible for my initial entry into the business world. However, in the past few years I have worn glasses instead of contact lenses to look more serious and intellectual. I used my looks to get my foot in the door and then hoped my intelligence would show through in the interview. I did that in my early 30s; it's disgusting, but it worked. I can't understand women who seriously play the "cute" game, however. I know women do it but at the same time I don't want to know.

Women have had the biggest effect on my professional life; as a matter of fact, I have never had a male boss. One of the women I worked with several years ago was very demanding and always threw people into the most awkward situations. She often gave me just five minutes' notice to present a set of slides in a meeting. And each time, I got so sick I ended up in the bathroom with diarrhea, wasting my precious preparation time. But I always did the best I could. At the time I resented her methods tremendously and thought she was awful, but in the end she really helped me by her dramatic mentoring. It was a sick thing for her to do but I survived and learned a lot from her.

I have few friends professionally or socially. I'm most comfortable with one-on-one relationships. I can count on one hand the people I'm close to. I never joined groups, participated in anything, or played on any teams in college. I'm like that in business, too.

I've decided that when I take my next job, I will start off differently. I won't make the same mistakes I made before. I want to be more organized and start out with the best clothes I can afford. Full armor, as they say. If I wear my best business suits, I'll feel better and do a better job. I'll be more comfortable and look the part. I don't want anything to show through that shouldn't show through. The more layers I put on, the less people can get to me.

The move from one town to another in fifth grade undermined me badly and left me feeling very insecure. That's one reason I would never go back to another high school reunion. I went back for my tenth, and even though I looked my best then, I still felt I was regressing back to high school days. Here I was a wonderful, accomplished person with a great career making a good salary, and I felt just like little old weak me. Now my twentieth reunion is coming up but it would just bring back all those same insecurities. I have tried to tell myself that I haven't peaked yet and it was better that my successes came later in life. But I still think I'll take a pass on the twentieth reunion.

I've always said that I didn't mind getting older because I never valued my looks as much as my intelligence anyway. It's not getting older that bothers me. What bothers me is the feeling that I should have accomplished more by this point.

JOYCE, 48:
music teacher, supervisor

My memories of my appearance as a child are extremely negative. I guess there was a brief time when I was very small that people said I was cute. However, when I started school I never felt like the other kids. I had very straggly hair, and in kindergarten I had to have glasses. They were little round glasses that are popular now, but they were ugly then. And that was terrible—that just added to it! All the way through grade school, I tried so hard to do different things with my hair and my clothes, and I just think that I always looked like a loser. I had nice friends; I was always with a group. But I always felt like I was on the fringe.

Part of it was that my mother didn't know how to do some of these things. She didn't know how to fix hair. She would give us a perm and it would be just terrible. I have to say that my sister didn't look any better than I did, so I had company.

That would sum up my childhood pretty well. I never felt really attractive and I never felt that the boys thought I was cute. And apparently they didn't. I didn't have a lot of boyfriends and the girls in my school started with boyfriends quite young then—in fifth, sixth, seventh grade.

From kindergarten all the way through eighth grade, I lived in the shadow of another little girl in the neighborhood who came from a family that had a lot more money and did fancier things. Although we were both very small, she was very cute. It didn't matter what she wore or how she fixed her hair, she always looked cute. And I felt just the opposite. No matter what I did, I didn't look cute.

I don't know that anything my parents or siblings did or said really influenced the way I felt about myself. My brother always treated me like a little sister; I think he thought I was cute. I certainly wasn't bizarre looking, but I just didn't feel good about myself.

During the teenage years, I had a lot of friends but it was more my personality that attracted them. I started to blossom a little bit with a good sense of humor. I know I definitely looked better in high school. I started learning how to take care of my hair which was quite nice by then. And I always had a nice complexion. I wasn't obsessed, but I was always concerned about how I looked.

Whether it made a big difference to other people, I don't know, but when I got into college I got contact lenses. That had been my dream! Then I could do more things with my hair without the stigma of glasses. I let my hair grow very long. I'd pile it up, or just leave it down. For a couple of years I was very, very popular. I realized that I was very attractive at that time. I probably even got a little cocky about it! That's okay. I deserved it. From then, I continued to feel good about my looks well into adulthood.

In college, I had a lot of boyfriends. I know they were attracted primarily by my looks, and the fact that they came around made me feel good about myself. And when, as a young adult working in California, I met Robert, my ex-husband, he just went gah-gah! I think that's what I liked— the fact that he really thought I was something else.

I kept my hair long for quite a while, even after I had my children. Finally I decided it would be more in keeping with my age to cut it, not because I was old but because long hair was a thing of the past. So I have gone with shorter hair. I have always had this fear of going bald, because I have very thin, very fine hair. I was always looking in the mirror for any bald spots! I still want to look nice, but I'm not as concerned as I was when I was younger.

I am divorced, not dating now, and have no immediate intentions in that direction, but I don't think I'd get real hung up on how I look. I would dress up, but if someone were attracted to me and I were attracted to him, I don't think I would go out of my way to change my appearance. "This is the way I look. I think I look good. You better think I look good, too, or it's your loss!"

I've come to realize that looks aren't everything. There was that one stage in college when I was a very, very pretty girl; I knew people looked when I walked by and I liked that. Now when I think of my appearance, I think of all of me—my personality and everything that goes into the way I look, even my mannerisms. People are attracted to me. Maybe that's a good word—attractive—not pretty, not beautiful. But because of all my aspects put together, I think people do find me attractive, not just because of my face or my hair but the whole thing. And I am kinda cute, anyway!

I was prettier at a younger age, but I think I feel better about my looks now. I was so obsessed with my looks then that maybe I didn't enjoy them as much as I could have. Yeah, I feel good. First thing in the morning sometimes is a real shocker, but I'm satisfied with the way I look now. And it's a good feeling to be comfortable with myself.

If my appearance ranked equally with my intellect, I'd really be gorgeous! I have a lot going for me: personality, achievement, intellect! I think appearance could improve in order to stay equal with those other factors! But now it's not that important to me. I'm sure there is a gap between the mirror image and the self-image. People will read this and then see what I look like and say, "Holy Toledo, is she blind in both eyes or just one?" I'm sure there's a gap, but that doesn't matter. Sometimes I don't even look in the mirror. I just figure I look okay and off I go.

Some of the people I care about most are my young music students, and many of them, day after day, tell me, "You look pretty today. I like what you are wearing. I like the way you look all over today." That makes me feel good, because they are the people I work with and the ones I'm dressing for, besides myself. They are very responsive. It gives me a nice feeling and it's so cute, especially from the little ones. They will all raise their hands at once, and look like they are going to tell me something momentous or announce they have to throw up. And I will say, "What do you need?" And this little voice says, "You look pretty today, teacher!" And I usually say something like, "Thank you for mentioning it." It always gives me a nice feeling.

These days I wear clothes that I probably wouldn't wear if I weren't working with young children. I have sweaters with large cats with glittery eyes that say "Cool Cats!" I often wear earrings in the shape of little, fuzzy pink pigs or large cats that hang down and do strange things. And that's kind of fun! It's a wonderful way to dress with kids. It's very stimulating and entertaining for them. Occasionally if I go to the bank or to see my lawyer after work, I find him staring at my ears. And then I realize that I am wearing those fuzzy, pink pig earrings, and he will comment on how interesting my earrings are: "Are those pigs?" "Yes, they sure are! You ought to see the cats I have, or the orange spider webs, with black spiders crawling up them. And the reindeers with googlie eyes are some of the best!"

The kids make me feel good and encourage me to wear things that are more outlandish. I used to be very, very conservative for school. But I've worked with a lot of student teachers in the past few years, many of whom are extremely heavy and yet wear bright purple dresses with colorful scarves and wild jewelry. And here I am 110 pounds soaking wet, and I am wearing my little beige sweater and beige pants. But now I have my pig earrings!

I think I am as happy as I can be with the way I look. There's not a lot I can do to change it. I am always going to have fine, thin hair and be restricted in what I can do with it. I see a few little wrinkles and sags, and I'm not too happy about it, but it's not something of great concern to me. The one thing that really bothers me is saggy arms, especially if someone comes up and grabs me by the arm. So, a couple summers ago, I started lifting small weights on my own. I've been walking for about six or seven years, and I also started running, but the people in the neighborhood were collapsing in laughter! They said they had never seen anybody run so slow, and sweat so much! So I cut back to walking. But in the winter, I don't walk as much, so the old thunder thighs' reappearance means I have to get at it again in the spring. That bothers me. And I do get concerned about getting fat because I am so short. I'm not anywhere near fat, but I am a little blubbery or untoned, so I work on that.

I don't see myself making any great changes, though. I worry that I may not be able to wear my contact lenses after a while. I guess that goes all the way back to kindergarten and my first pair of glasses. I see other people wearing glasses and they look great. But I don't like mine. I have such a heavy prescription that they just don't look nice on me. But if that time comes, I'll work on it.

Dealing with the aging process? Well, I've got stock in Oil of Olay and Avon! It's funny, when I think of old people, I think of my mother's looks and I don't want to look like that. I may look sort of like that, but I'll never look exactly like that. It's okay for her; she's 80 years old and she's supposed to look like that. I say I won't! But of course I will. I hope it doesn't become a real issue with me. There are so many other things that are important, but when it starts happening, you sing another tune. I guess I'll just go with it. There's not much I can do.

K Y L E, 30:
fashion designer

My most distinct memory of my appearance is from junior high. Prior to that I don't remember any strong feedback either way, so I always considered myself as average-looking. Not ugly, not pretty, not exceptional in any way, just average. But in junior high, one of my friends told me that her mother said I was homely; that shook my cage. I thought, "You mean all these years I thought I was average and I was actually homely?" That comment will stick in my memory for the rest of my life. Not that I agree or disagree with the woman's perception, but she should never have done that to a youngster.

I don't remember much more than that one incident regarding my physical appearance. I strove to do well in academics, music, and creative things and didn't really see how my looks made a big difference. So even though that woman said I was homely, it didn't change anything in my life or my goals. I didn't think about appearance stuff much at all, so it's strange that I ended up in the fashion business where appearances are so important.

I remember a photograph of a very pretty lady on a table at my grandma's house when I was very small. When I asked about it, Grandma said it was my mom's cousin: it was her high school graduation picture and she was the valedictorian. So I found out at a very young age what a valedictorian was and I wanted to be like her, to accomplish what she accomplished. I wanted to be in that picture frame. Even in early grade school that was my goal. I was so young when I made that decision. Talk about driven!

The summer between sixth and seventh grade, at age 12, I got braces. My teeth where a little crooked and I wanted to get them taken care of as quickly as possible. I was one of the younger orthodontic kids at my school. My mom had worn braces; so had my sister. It was an important family thing.

I got teased a lot because I always had short hair. But that didn't bother me because I wanted short hair; I am a short-hair person. I would just laugh at the kids when they teased me. They called me all sorts of strange things, but that was okay.

The friend who claimed her mother said I was homely had the biggest negative impact on me during my earlier years. Having just seen her at a class reunion a year ago, I realize now how delicate her self-esteem is. In some way she must have been threatened by me; of course, that didn't occur to me at the time. It was a given that she was better than I was in everything. I hung out with her because she was the only one in my league of academic goals. She wanted to get straight A's as much as I did, so we studied together; that was the basis for our friendship. In retrospect, I wouldn't call her a close friend. Only since graduating from college have I really developed close friends. Everyone else was just an acquaintance by comparison. Some of my current friends are so positive and helpful—like friends are supposed to be.

I am pretty strong-willed. I usually know what I want and I have an opinion about most things. And there were some incidents throughout school when I was shamed by the teachers for something I said. If I offered an alternative method or plan, sometimes they didn't want to hear it. I am sure I set them on edge. It wasn't that I was bad, or had bad intentions. But, again, it's a terrible thing for an adult to do to a child.

I will never forget being shamed in first grade. I raised my hand innocently, made a suggestion, and the teacher humiliated me by reprimanding me in front of the whole class. I cried for hours. It was nothing to her, but it was a big thing for me. In retrospect, I know the teacher wanted to remain in control of the class; however, situations like that which used to be common can be damaging for kids, especially at such a tender age.

My mother is currently doing a lot of work with experimental educational methods in Minnesota, where the educational system is very progressive. Educators are learning some valuable things now about socializing children, and it's about time. Much of it has to do with children who are extremely creative. I put myself in that category; some of my teachers didn't know what to do with me. It's obvious to me now that the situation in first grade was the teacher's only way of dealing with me. I am sure she was freaked out. But then there were other teachers who saw me as an opportunity, a challenge, a chance to experiment with different ways of thinking. I know I was way out there sometimes, but my family never discouraged that behavior.

My family and relatives must have been very positive in terms of my self-image because I don't remember anything negative. I didn't feel held back or thwarted or redirected. It couldn't have been an issue to me at the time; I was too busy pursuing all of my interests. In high school I was very involved in a small musical group of 20 to 25 kids that performed many times during the year. When I wasn't studying, I was practicing and performing all the time which was a tremendous experience.

My concept of my appearance during teenage years and high school was that I was average. I didn't think about my looks, and I'm glad I didn't put any more emphasis on them; that would only have gotten in my way. In my late teens and 20s, it felt weird to hear people say I was pretty. Where I grew up, on a farm, the whole environment is not one of first impressions. But the small city where I attended a liberal arts college, majoring in home economics/fashion design, was an environment where first impressions were important. People remembered me and said, "You're the pretty one." That was remarkable to me! I was used to being recognized for my accomplishments.

In early adulthood, when I started hearing the words "pretty" or "attractive," I began to realize the impact of my appearance. I had done some modeling in college for a fashion show and had received a lot of positive feedback. That surprised me, but it didn't occur to me that the feedback had anything to do with my looks. I was simply performing a task.

At one of my first jobs, however, being pretty was such a problem that it ended my employment. Although I was hired as a designer, I think the company really wanted a pretty young girl to accompany the salesmen for presentations. Well, it didn't register with me at first; I was only 22 years old. Unfortunately all I was meant to do was look good and smile. They didn't want me for anything else and I didn't want to be there for that. It was a problem. I still think they were really stupid but it was a misinterpretation on both sides. There were stories about how promiscuous I was—absolutely contrary to reality—because the salesmen just didn't like the fact that I wouldn't play the game. I was so insulted. How could they have such a warped sense of a female? How could they be so disrespectful? I guess they just didn't know any better. The funny thing is, the woman who replaced me won a sexual harassment suit against the company! So I was vindicated; I wasn't crazy. If only I had had the wherewithal to do something about it sooner. That was a memorable experience and one reason to become an entrepreneur—to get out of that environment.

If I could have applied what I know now to my appearance five years ago, things would have been different; maybe things would have been different at all the jobs I've held since college. I can see now why certain things happened and I would have quit that infamous job even faster. But it was a very valuable learning experience.

One of my male friends had a big impact on me during the time I was learning to deal with the fact that men thought I was pretty. Prior to meeting him, I had no idea the male perspective was different. My dad and all the men I grew up with had operated on a performance scale: "Boy, Kyle, you can really cook up a wicked bucket of stew! You are really musically inclined!" Stuff like that. But this particular male was a true friend. We didn't have a dating relationship, but he made a big difference because he was the first male peer to give me a lot of validation for personal qualities like intuition and spirituality, making my appearance a side issue and just a part of the package. His opinion was that everybody has a package and whatever it is, the person had better learn to work with it. He gave me permission to be okay with myself and to pursue people who recognized my entire package, not just my looks. I really listened to what he said.

I consciously tried to counteract the discomfort of men coming on to me sexually and I still do that. In college I carried an extra 20 or 30 pounds. I didn't want to hear those come-ons and I screened out some of it that way. It's only been in the past four or five years that I have gotten rid of the weight—and that was because the man I dated at the time didn't care if I had extra weight. Figuring out if I *wanted* the weight or not was very different than making sure I had it. And when it didn't matter how much I weighed, I quit weighing myself. What mattered was how I felt; if I felt healthy and strong that's what was important.

I just turned 30 this year and it was a big deal for me. I decided that this is the time to start figuring out how I want things. The most important thing for me right now is to be recognized as a professional. The way I look at my job, at creative projects, the way I dress, and whether I put on makeup or not are all coming into a very different perspective. Because I am in the fashion business, I am looking at my image as a tool now more than ever before. Although I deal with my clients' image on an individual basis every day, I had never understood what I was working with, but now I look at myself as a client, too. I constantly ask myself, "Where are you going? What are your intentions? How do you want to be perceived?" I am really digging into myself more than before, and it's a very interesting process.

I want to maintain the way my look evolves, but I want to be sure that I put myself together comfortably. Comfort is my main emphasis and not visual impact. That also goes for my personality. I am very practical and into things that work. I am not glamorous but I do like the element of glamour. It's one of the reasons I design. My main mistake in putting myself together may have been underdressing on purpose. My personal style is simple, classic, and minimal. Appropriateness and comfort, rather than visual impact, are my main emphasis. It's important that I look professional.

The term "professional" keeps coming to mind as my way of describing myself: respectable, with simple, elegant, classic style. Graceful. Natural beauty, including physical characteristics. I describe my physical self as attractive, healthy, fresh, and handsome. I would love other people to describe me as handsome. I use that word and I like it. Of course, people always say I look wholesome! I think I look better now than I did when I was younger. Or maybe I just have more peace of mind; that's a big factor in liking your looks.

I would say that my appearance qualifies as sometimes equal to and sometimes less than my personality and my achievement. I am happier when it's less; I feel stronger when my attention is not on my looks. At this point there isn't much of a gap between my mirror image and my self-image. I really don't mind looking at myself in the mirror, and I think I know how I look: better now than ever, but it varies from day to day, obviously.

I am not sure how most people perceive me. I think many people stop with my looks; not everyone is inclined pursue my real self. My close friends and I are all into personal growth and development, so we give each other much feedback. I am learning more about how others see me as part of being recognized as a professional. The things that I am recognized for have been fairly consistent, and that's nice to hear.

I am pretty happy with myself right now. I don't know of any changes that I need or want to make at this point. They will happen when they need to happen. I haven't actually given the aging process much thought. I do know that it's important to take care of myself: exercise, take care of my skin, and stay healthy. That's the best I can do. It has always bothered me that people think I am younger than I am. It used to be a real disadvantage. I'm okay with it now, but I wonder when it will flip.

I don't know if it was my family culture or the farm environment, but there was never an emphasis on getting a job. I have never heard that from my parents. My dad's advice was, "It doesn't matter what you do as long as you enjoy it. If you want to sell hotdogs, go ahead. You'll like it some days, hate it some days. But if you start out liking it, you have a better chance." That was the only career advice I got and that was after I was out of college. It was never that I had to get the "right" job, or a "good paying" job, or have a "career."

I recently had a wonderful learning experience in a class on drum making. The teacher was really invisible as a teacher, facilitating rather than taking center stage. The class was not at all about him; he didn't get in our way! I loved that. He was the way all of my teachers should have been. I was able to feel good about learning, not feel bad about doing it wrong!

L E I G H, 48:
real-estate appraiser

As a little girl I remember looking like the Dutch Boy Cleanser ad with very straight hair and a bowl haircut. All four of us girls had the same haircut, which was very unattractive in my opinion. In addition to that, Mother used to make us all wear brown socks and brown oxfords! She said they went with pants and with skirts and it didn't make any difference. Although I didn't like them, they didn't really make me feel bad; I just thought they were ugly.

At age 10, I got loafers and could jettison the oxfords as a rite of passage. Because I'm the oldest of four girls, I felt I had to break away from those styles for the sake of my younger sisters. So, for each of my sisters, the advent of the loafers got a little sooner. I was first and had to convince my mom that my little sisters should get them. I had been embarrassed and weathered it, but I was more embarrassed for my sisters than for myself.

We used to kid my mom about those brown shoes and socks and tell her how awful it was. And she said, "Well, it was the easiest way to do it with four kids." My father was very strict and when he said do it, you did it. And of course there were no fights over the best shoes; we all had the same ones. At that younger age we didn't care much, but those oxfords gradually gained mythic proportions in our family.

My father used to get very angry with my next younger sister Chris, for being an independent thinker and speaking her mind. She wouldn't toe the line. I knew how to play the game, and that's how I perceived myself— as knowing when to do things and when not. It's safe that way. My sister never wanted to be safe; she always bucked the system and always got punished for it. I watched and learned from that. I was never real gutsy; I just lived the way I was directed by my parents. My sister's experiences helped me learn how to get along even better.

As for physical traits, all I can remember was my god-awful straight hair. All I wanted was curly hair! I remember my grandmother giving me a perm: the ends were straight but it was all kinky in the middle. It was hopeless, so she cut it off again, even shorter. It looked awful.

In terms of personality traits, I was very self-satisfied. I went along, didn't ruffle any feathers, and just grew up. I don't remember being terribly unhappy. As I got older, I used to get angry with my parents' tunnel vision about some things but as a little girl I had a good time. I took my mom's peanut butter and jelly sandwiches—with olives planted on top—to school for lunch everyday and thought they were delicious.

My maternal grandmother was a lovely and sophisticated lady who would take me and my cousin June, who is six days younger than I am, and dress us up and parade us wherever she wanted. She would buy us the exact same dress, one in pink and one in blue. June and I went to visit her a lot. My grandfather travelled regularly so he would often fly us down to Florida to keep her company. She loved our visits.

My grandmother was the one relative who affected my self-image by making me feel special. And my cousin felt the same way. This special treatment carried all the way through college; June and I were always the ones invited to go to Florida. My sisters never got that, and I'm sure they felt slighted. It was an unspoken thing. But it wasn't favoritism towards me, because my cousin was treated the same way, and she and I were good friends. It was because there were no other real close cousins on either side.

My very strict father always said that parents and children had their own places; a child was to be seen and not heard. He also felt strongly that girls were no less important than boys, and needed four years of college. My grandfather, on the other hand, believed that girls needed no more than two years of college; they didn't need a degree.

My father always expected his daughters to do what he thought. And although the rest of us did what he expected of us, Chris fought it. My parents didn't have expectations that we would be president or a corporate chairman, but that we would go for our potential, do what made us happy, and at the same time make them proud of us. We were all brought up that way.

In the teen years and high school, I had a good time: I did everything in high school I wanted to do. My feelings about myself were positive. I wasn't the cutesy, bubbly, cheerleader type, but I had dates and I was on the homecoming court. I was a little reserved; I would have liked to have been more outgoing but it wasn't in my personality at the time.

I was tall, thin, and short-waisted. I looked fine but I just didn't look like the cute, 5'2" cheerleader type. Being tall, per se, was never really an issue, but I always wondered why the tall basketball players dated those little short girls! I always ended up going to a dance with someone who was just my height. In a pair of heels I was usually taller than my date because some of the high school boys hadn't grown yet.

I got a lot of positive reinforcement in high school; as a result, I was very confident. I was president of my sorority. I was doing things all along. When our high school basketball team and cheerleaders went to the state tournament, I was chosen to represent our high school on the State of Illinois court with girls from all the other schools. I was on TV and had a couple of pictures in the newspaper. That experience had a strong impact on me. Those four years were a growing experience, so by the time I was a senior I felt pretty well-rounded.

My college years constituted young adulthood; I had more fun in college than in high school. I was a little more serious in high school while under the control of my parents, but I had always loved being away from home, especially going away to camp during summers while growing up. So of course I went away to college, to a big state university where I didn't know anybody.

I had come from a town that, at the time, was small. My family on both my parents' sides were long-time residents in that town. They didn't have a lot of money, but they were well known, so I was always so-and-so's daughter. When I went away to school, I wanted to be out on my own and not be so-and-so's daughter; I wanted to succeed on my own merits.

I went through Rush Week even though I didn't know much about it. The sorority I selected was not one of the three my dad had recommended when he urged me to rush, but I did just fine. I was where I wanted to be, and my friends were great. I made my own college experience.

I dated a lot my freshman year; then I was pinned to a guy who was at school in the East. I had dated him for a year and a half when our relationship blew up. So for a while my self-image went down, but then I got back into the dating scene again. By the time I graduated, I was dating John, my future husband, regularly and exclusively.

I earned a bachelor's degree in History and English and couldn't do a darn thing, so my father said, "You need to get your teaching certificate." For a year after I graduated, I lived at home and worked afternoons for an insurance company, while going to school in the mornings. At the end of the year when I got my teaching certificate John and I got engaged and then married. That was my young adulthood!

I taught for only two years. I was married in 1966, and our daughter was born in 1968. Young adulthood was being a married lady—not too many exciting events, but I was very happy. John and I had a good time. All those first things: buying a house, doing the whole process.

I have evolved. Back then I wasn't really my own person. I didn't want to be and I didn't try to be. I am much more confident about myself than I was back then. I feel better with age and experience.

My husband is THE special man in my life; we are a good compliment to each other. My father was special, in his own way. And I had a wonderful grandfather who was also important in my life. The guy I went with in college didn't have much impact on my self-image ultimately. There were guys in high school and college who made me feel special because they liked me and wanted to go out with me—not because of the way I looked, but because we were friends.

I have a lot of women friends but I don't know that they have had that much impact on my self-image—other than one friend from my hometown. She and I are still very good friends. I just think that all good friendships are positive things. It makes you feel good and therefore you look good, as good as you are given to look.

I haven't made any major changes in my self-image; I have simply grown stronger and more self-assured from experience. And I haven't had any real major disappointments in my life. If my marriage blew up, that would undermine my self-worth. I've had disappointments: the loss of a parent, a child's major medical problem, and the fact that I couldn't have any more children of my own. But for the most part, things have gone well in my life, and I am pretty positive about my life and myself. Every day adds a little more stress or tension, of course. Kids throw you into another dimension. But at this point I have to step back and say, "I did the best I could, and if it's wrong, who knows."

Once I got past the bowl-cut hair and the brown shoes, I felt positive enough about myself. I didn't like being short-waisted, and I've always had a long, pointed nose which preempted a lot of nose-accentuating hairstyles. When I was pregnant and the weather was hot, I'd pull my long hair back and John would tell me I looked like George Washington. Or he'd say my nose was getting more pointed! Some of my features are just not wonderful—things that I could program myself to be unhappy about. But I do have long legs and small hands, which are positive things in my view. I hate having my father's big, bulgy eyes with shadows under them, but I can't change them, and it doesn't negate my self-image.

No, I don't think I look better than ever at the present. I honestly think we all look the best between 25 and 40-something. I would describe myself as pleasing, comfortable, attractive. A lot of people are attractive even if they aren't beautiful or pretty, depending on how they present themselves. It comes from inside, or from what they've done with their wardrobe, or what they've done with what they've got to work with. I guess attractive would probably be the best word for me to use to describe myself. Most people I know are attractive, nice looking, well put together.

For a long time, I have known that I work well with people and people work well with me. I have always enjoyed the group projects sponsored by the organizations I've joined; I have always been very lucky that co-workers have been very supportive. When I am asked to head a project, it's a compliment to my capabilities; when someone completes a project I've asked them to do it's a compliment to my leadership abilities. Maybe it's not a true verbal compliment, but I take it as a compliment.

I am happy with myself today, and I don't see a gap between my self-perceptions and the way others see me. Growing old doesn't scare or bother me, nor does aging or my appearance. In ten years I'll be 60; that is scary because my mom died at 64. The closer I get to it, the younger it seems. Fourteen years is such a short time. And I don't really want to leave that soon—not that I have a choice. But that scares me more than my physical appearance or anything else about aging. I just hope I have my health. I don't want to be in a wheelchair, or end up with hips and knees that don't work, or become a crotchety old lady sitting in her house. I have always said that if I reach 80, they can take me anytime after that. I'd like to be in my 80s and still be active—walking, talking, thinking clearly—and just go in my sleep like my grandmother did.

The idea of a nursing home scares me more than an aging appearance. As long as I can function, that's the most important thing. John would never come to visit me in a nursing home; he just hates them. He said to me, "Don't you ever put me in one of those places! When I get bad, just put me in my wheelchair on top of the boathouse, and shove me off into the lake! In the north woods, in the fresh air, and with nature." Well, that's easy for him to say.

One of our friends developed Alzheimer's and her husband went to visit her in the nursing home every day for years as she got worse and worse. John said he could never handle something like that, and I don't think he could. Well, if John won't take care of me, I'll have to look to my friends! They can come and take me out to the boathouse!

L E N A, 58:
retired retail buyer

The first memory I have of my appearance as a child was when I made my confirmation at age 11. My professional photograph made me look much taller and thinner, which was what I wanted to be. However, I had not realized what a dark complexion I had, until I saw myself against my stark white dress. I didn't think I was very pretty.

From the time I was able to understand, I always believed that I was a short, fat little girl. My family always called me fat. But as time went on, I realized I wasn't a short, fat little girl but a rather pretty child, based on the compliments I received about my physical appearance, my eyes, my round face, my small nose.

My sisters, however, continued to call me fat and constantly reminded me that I had short, fat legs. From the time I was about 10 months old until I was 6 1/2, I wore braces to straighten out my badly bowed legs. Growing up, I realized that I had some attractive features that my sisters didn't have; however, I've always been sensitive about my legs. Even though they were straightened, they were always short and heavy. To this day they are the bane of my existence.

Looking back, I realize that I was a prettily dressed child until the age of 3, because my godfather constantly gave me beautiful clothes. After that, I wore hand-me-downs. But during those three years, I looked extremely pretty.

As I continued to grow, I developed a much better self-image, because by the age of 16 and with my first part-time job, I was able to select and pay for all my own clothing. I learned a great deal about coordinating clothing and makeup and also about styling my hair. I had a good head of hair and I was able to pay to have it styled frequently.

I was also able to improve my hands. I had always been told that they were short and stubby, and because I did so much housework as a kid, I had chapped hands and broken nails. But when I started working and getting my nails done professionally on a regular basis, I found I had very expressive hands. Even though they were not the long, slender hands most people think of as beautiful, they were and still are very arresting and expressive. I take good care of my hands because I learned through compliments that they are one of my finer physical characteristics. People often think that expression is only in the face and the eyes but, being of Italian background, I cannot talk unless my hands are moving. And in expressing myself and knowing that I have physically attractive hands, I use them as much as possible to show my pride in this particular physical attribute!

I was also sensitive about the appearance of my teeth. As a child, I had some broken teeth which could not be fixed at the time for financial reasons. I had them repaired when I grew older, but I feel very strongly that they always affected my ability to smile. Even though I may feel happy within, I am unable to smile comfortably because my front teeth were particularly unattractive during the formative years.

While I was growing up, my parents, relatives, and especially my sisters, found it very difficult to ever tell me that I looked nice or that I was pretty. Even as an adult, when I would get dressed up and ask them how I looked, they would be very negative. That has left a mark on me; however, I have come to consider it "professional jealousy!"

I have three brothers, wonderful people, who also found it very difficult to ever compliment their baby sister on anything. They would do it with strangers, but not with me, and I think they shared my parents' attitude that compliments were to come from outside the family.

Even though I'm sure my mother believed that I was attractive, she always reminded me that it was not a mother's duty to tell me that I was pretty; it was up to other people to compliment her children, not her. She believed in the Italian superstition that if compliments were paid, an evil spirit would come upon the recipient. But when I was older, and the rest of my brothers and sisters had married and moved out, I think my mother finally came to see me as attractive.

When I got into high school, got a job, and was able to buy my own wardrobe, I received good feedback from some of my closer friends who said nice things about my appearance and my clothes. This never happened in my family, however.

The fact that my finances were limited in high school, that I was responsible for buying my own clothes, and also that my mother's trade was tailoring, taught me that it was best to buy quality. That way I would have serviceable and wearable clothing for a long period of time. I learned to select good fabric over fashion and I stayed very close to the basics. Today, even though I have the means, I am extremely careful when selecting clothes. I want good looks and long-term serviceability, and I am also very concerned about price. Quality has to come with the price, as far as I am concerned!

During my young adulthood, I was earning enough to purchase not only quality but also fashion. I deprived myself of other things, and put most of my money and time into clothes. Therefore I feel I've developed a good sense of both fashion and quality. By the time I was out of school and working full time, I was spending a lot of money on my clothes and getting good feedback from my special friends for my fashionable image.

Another of my special interests is jewelry. I look at it not only as part of a costume but as an art form. Today, I have a great love of silver, as well as handcrafted or very creative jewelry. Like clothes, I acquired few pieces but of good quality, and I now have quite an extensive collection.

My self-image has changed a great deal over the past years. Because I literally grew up in the business world, I acquired a certain professional attitude toward dressing. Working my way up to a responsible position as a retail chain store buyer gave me the opportunity to learn to purchase and wear clothing that fit in very well with both my business and social life. Today, after many years of developing an extensive wardrobe of professional clothes, I have found that in retirement I no longer have the need for the same type of clothes. Therefore, I am gradually changing my wardrobe again into a still-conservative but more relaxed and comfortable style more suited to my casual lifestyle.

Of course, my self-image has changed a great deal since high school, not only because of my experiences in the business world but also because of major changes in my lifestyle over the years. I was born and grew up in Chicago, but my career allowed me to live and work and play in New York City. There I learned to understand more of life and to appreciate different lifestyles. I became very interested in the arts and in travel. I have experienced a tremendous amount of personal growth. This, of course, I attribute to my experiences and responsibilities in the business world, and the opportunities given to me along the way. They opened my eyes and my heart to many important aspects of life and helped keep me abreast of fashion, business, and the social and entertainment worlds.

Once when I was only about 8, some *pisans*, friends from an adjacent neighborhood, came unannounced to our house to visit. It was a woman friend of my mother's and her young daughter, who was about my age. I was so excited; here was a little girl, someone other than a relative to meet, play with, and get to know! I wanted them to stay so I could play with this new girl! I ran all the way to the grocery store to fetch my mother so she would spend time visiting with the woman and I could get to know this little girl. The only thing my mother could say to me all the way home was, "Stop jumping around and fidgeting, just carry those groceries, and behave yourself, calm down. Did you do your chores? If you didn't do your chores, you'll be in trouble." And all the way home she complained bitterly about these unexpected visitors.

When we got home, she sent me to finish my chores. The woman and her daughter stayed only a short time, and then they went home. I never got to meet the girl, or play with her or get to know her. I was so disappointed! This story always reminds me of how my little-girl enthusiasm got squelched. My parents insisted on responsible behavior from their children—no smiling, laughing, playing, or having fun. It wasn't until many years later that I found some of that childlike enthusiasm again when I went to live in New York. I was away from my family, and there was so much to see and do and be enthusiastic about! I also realized that I lost that enthusiasm again when I left New York and came back to live in Chicago near my family. I have managed to get back in touch with it only sporadically, and most often when I am on vacation, especially in a foreign country.

My time in New York gave me the chance to really appreciate my personal growth and the more positive thinking that I developed toward myself. I think the words that best describe my most positive mental image are: sophisticated, European-looking, knowledgeable, very responsible, and very loyal. Unlike the typical all-American girl, I did not possess the blonde hair, the blue eyes, and the natural beauty. However, I could in a sense stand out in the crowd because I did have some great ethnic features that set me apart from the rest: my high cheekbones, my long neck, my dark eyes, and my hands. So I portray myself as a European type. My looks have changed very little up until the past ten years; I have always had a rather young-looking face. But even now the onset of wrinkles brings out some of my better features, such as my cheekbones and my eyes. And I think I feel as attractive as I did when I was younger.

Today I perceive myself as a very accomplished individual. I managed to excel in the business world during a time when women were not afforded many opportunities. That allowed me to develop my personality, my intelligence, and my sense of responsibility. My accomplishments were numerous and I am very grateful for them. I see no gap between my self-image and my mirror image.

Contributing to my achievements in the business world was the fact that I take great pride in my reputation for being honest, personable, ambitious, and extremely hardworking. So to sum it up, I perceive myself as a pretty good kid! And now I can smile when I say that!

I think others perceive me as being honest. It's not very difficult to know what I am thinking because my facial expressions tell all. In the business world, I was frequently told by people that I was difficult to work with because I was so frank and honest, but I accept that as a compliment. There have also been times when I felt that people expected more of me than I expected of myself, or more than I thought I could produce, because I did not see my true value.

One of the major things that happened to me in business was being given the responsibility to develop projects and products. However, no one ever commented or complimented me on the results. That always left me with the feeling that what I had accomplished was unimportant and insignificant. Finally, I realized that the people to whom I was responsible never bothered to discuss a project with me because they knew I had the ability to do it. Deep down inside, I didn't feel I was accomplishing much—and because I was never questioned about any of the multimillion-dollar decisions I made, I thought they weren't important. It took me a long time to realize that I had the ability to do things without the direction of anyone other than myself. I had continued to feel insignificant because I was not getting the positive feedback I thought I needed to hear. It has not been until recently that I really began to appreciate my accomplishments. This has accounted for a gap between others' perceptions and my own.

Today, even after all my accomplishments, which brought a great deal of joy to me and to others, I would like to be able to express my happiness by smiling and laughing more easily. I continue to do some self-analysis. I think I can go back and draw from my experiences and truly apply what I have learned to my life today. I think the thing that makes me unhappy right now is not having the high-powered job which I held for so many years or any projects to be directly responsible for. I find it difficult to just enjoy people and do my own thing without feeling guilty for not accomplishing something. I have lived such a structured life for so long that I don't know what it's like to be relaxed. And one of the greatest things would be to express myself more openly with my facial features. I would like to be able to better express what I feel inside when I am happy, particularly with smiles. That would be a real accomplishment for me.

I don't have any difficulties dealing with the aging process, because I'm never going to get old! I am a great believer that age is a frame of mind. Some of us are fortunate enough to look younger longer than others. And when the day comes that I begin to show my age, I'm going to solicit the assistance of a few plastic surgeons, or whoever else! Maybe a diet, and liposuction. Back to the issue of my fat legs! I am smiling as I say that!

MARCIA, 40:
college student

The first memory I have of my appearance is from the age of 4 or 5. I had a lisp because my teeth were too big for my face, and an over-abundance of thick, black, curly hair. Combing my hair wasn't my mother's specialty, so just before kindergarten she took me to a beauty shop and had me sheared. That started my phobia about beauty shops: the smell was dreadful and I did not feel transformed. Rather, I was kind of ticked off; I wanted long hair. Cinderella, not Mary Martin, was my role model! Cinderella had long hair. Mary Martin had short hair. In all the fairy tales, the women had long tresses.

My mom kept my hair short until eighth grade, when I felt I was old enough to refuse to have it cut. After letting my hair grow out, I didn't cut it again until well into high school years; but the shorter length was only to my shoulders, so it wasn't really "cut." In those days, ethnic hair was not yet in style, so I ironed my very curly Semitic hair for a long time because even the professional straightening chemicals didn't work on me. I'll always remember going with my friend Blanca to the Spanish lady hairdresser to have my hair straightened, and it lasted for only one day. Now, everyone wants curly hair!

Everyone in my family always said my sister was the really beautiful one. Although we look very much alike, my sister was always cherished much more for her good looks. For a long time I also thought she was more attractive; now I am just aware of the similarities in our looks. People recognize us as sisters even though she is so much more petite than I am. Ah, yes, the dainty woman theory. She has small bones. I have average bones that belong to a taller person. For years I thought I had big hands and feet, until one day I realized I was in fact short. But everyone in my family was so short, that compared to them I was tall. That was a shock. I had thought I was a big woman, but I'm not.

Throughout eighth grade and freshman year in high school, I did the girl things: shaving my legs, wearing eyeliner and sneaking on more makeup than was allowed. I even had the perfect "flip" hairdo at last, thanks to the torment of sleeping with my hair rolled on orange juice can rollers. By the time I finished my sophomore year, I was an avid reader becoming more aware of national politics as well as women's emerging political issues. I was busy reading such things as *Our Bodies, Ourselves* and learning about the politics of female sexuality. Growing up in the Judaic tradition, where a woman's hair is considered to be sexual— Hasidic women wear wigs to cover their hair and yet they talk about the "crowning jewel"—you are made to feel that it is a lurid thing to have tresses. And at the same time people talk about "how beautiful your hair is, darling!"

My family culture was also full of mixed messages. It was the reverse of the norm for female behavior or even hypocritical. My mother said that girls should be seen and not heard, but in reality my father was quiet and withdrawn and my mother was in charge. She was the major breadwinner and she talked so much and so fast! She nattered! We were a loud family. Nobody talked at what would be considered a normal vocal tone. In our family the louder you spoke the better you'd be understood or the better your point would come across. So it took me a long time to learn to whisper. And then for a long time I talked very quietly.

After my sophomore year in high school, I made a conscious decision to dress a certain way. No teenager will ever admit to dressing to offend the universe, but they do: "Take me on my terms. If you don't like me, that's your problem." I was obnoxious about it, really! I didn't wear a bra, and if people looked at my breasts, I looked them in the eye and said, "Are you talking to me?" Plus, I had masses of curly hair, enough for three women. My mother always said, "Pull it back! You have a lovely face but we never get to see it!" That went on for years.

I was never invested in going to high school. There was art and theatre and music! I was one of the artsy-fartsy girls and I was concentrating on my artwork. At 19, my weight shot up to 165 pounds on my 5'3" frame. I was eating like a football player and doing theatre, *South Pacific*. I played Bloody Mary. I realized I had to lose that weight and by the time the show closed I was down to about 140 pounds. Then for a long time I hovered around 130, which is where I am now and which seems to be fine visually. Resolving some of these conflicting issues was the beginning of becoming very aware of how I looked and how I appeared to others.

Because of my theatre work, makeup became for me what you put on your face when you were on stage. For that reason, it seemed very unreal to wear makeup on a daily basis. It took me a very long time to come up with the concept that putting on a little lipstick and mascara was some-thing that other people could relate to. In the same way, I finally came to understand that polishing your nails is a sign of status and leisure. People always said, "you have such beautiful nails, you should let them grow out!" But then I wouldn't be able to garden or make pottery or art. That's a real contradiction in our culture. If women look purposeful, it can be detri-mental. It can be seen as not caring about personal appearance. On the other hand, all the feminine things women had always done to themselves were now beginning to be seen as negatives, because women were sacri-ficing who they were in order for people to accept them as embodiments of the feminine ideal.

It also took me a long time to relate positively to beauty shops, espe-cially after my childhood experiences of shearing. The first time I had my hair cut, as an adult, was at age 21. I had broken up with the love of my life, who had always talked about my long, beautiful hair. After that, I never really wanted my hair long again because I realized what a pain in the neck it was. Then for a long time, my co-workers in retail display cut my hair and dressed me. I dressed very artsy-fartsy because I was also a potter and in theatre. Both things helped shape my life.

Even as I reached young adulthood, I was still changing my focus and learning to play with my image. I later resolved some of my appearance conflicts while working at an advertising agency, where I learned a lot about image. As an artist, I was working in the paste-up room with glue and Xacto knives and other dirty stuff. I normally dressed for the mess in pants and junk stuff. But, once, in the very same week, I cut my wild mane of hair and wore a skirt to work. I will always remember that incident because people reacted so strongly to the change, as if I were a different person. Suddenly both men and women who hadn't previously talked to me were saying hello and chatting. To them I probably looked more normal, more like what they expected of a girl.

By the time I was 22 or 23, I realized all the things I had done in high school were taunting. Although at 23 I was wearying of my accustomed role, I was still testing everyone's patience and probably continued to do so until my late 20s.

A big change occurred when I realized I could get what I wanted because I knew what was expected of me. And that's not bad. I always thought that was manipulation because of the things the girls at school did to get what they wanted. I thought that was really disgusting. I never learned the fawning—do this to get this—kind of game. And I never wanted to be a princess. She doesn't get to be in charge. I always wanted to be queen. With the tiara, the big one! And it cracks me up, because that is what a lot of other women say.

When I really started playing with my image I was going out with a man who was really acculturated and very sensitive to design. He never made a thing about my appearance, but we talked about it and I began to change the way I thought. He would simply buy me something and say, "I thought this would look nice on you!" So I would try it on and maybe give it a chance. Also, as dance partners we were different enough yet close enough in size that we could mirror each other on the dance floor. I began to play with what was going on while we danced! I would look at him and he would look at me. He was half Indian and had very black hair. I had very black hair. And we both had these noses! It was very entertaining to be a part of that.

It still amazes me that people react so differently depending on what I am doing and how I am dressed. It is a game to me, and I use it in many ways. When I first started working as a sales associate in women's corporate apparel, I couldn't afford new clothes. My wardrobe consisted of 37 pairs of blue jeans and one dress. At first I wasn't going to put on the corporate costume just because people couldn't interpret me; then I began to look at it as an art project. Having already worked in display, I began to see clothing as something I could manipulate. Because I needed a professional wardrobe quickly, I started shopping at the good thrift shops. I knew the formulas for the corporate look as well as the color palette, so I could put the look together in thriftwear while I slowly invested in new clothes. I also knew a lot about fabric and construction, so buying used clothing actually gave me a better quality wardrobe along with the image I needed.

When I dressed appropriately to do a corporate clothing seminar, I was simply dressing to do a seminar, but my supervisors never understood that I didn't feel the need to dress that way for work every day. In fact it has taken a long time for those in the upper echelons of management to recognize my ability even after seeing me do a seminar. They don't understand that even though I can create the corporate look for my clients, I am not necessarily interested in producing that look for myself. The relevance of it for me is "only when it's necessary," as opposed to "it's necessary every day." Of course, it has given me a lot of insight into helping other women create the corporate look every day, because our culture teaches people that unless they look a certain way, unless they are a certain height or a certain weight, they aren't acceptable professionally or socially. Or to themselves.

I had vowed I would never get rid of my family nose like most of the other Jewish girls did when their families moved to the Jewish suburbs. When they turned 16, they got their choice of a car or a nose job! My parents weren't going to give me either a nose job (immoral) or a car (impossible).

However, because I had suffered from terrible migraine headaches and TMJ for many years, I began to consider facial surgery. I was an actress and doing a lot of auditioning, and wanted a more photogenic face. My face was noticeably asymmetrical, and though it wasn't displeasing, the change would give it more balance.

Part of me wanted to have the surgery, but the other part wasn't thrilled. It was the face I had had my whole life. Something inside me said, "Wait a minute! You want to let them break your face on purpose?"

It's still peculiar to me because it goes against all my feelings that it's wrong to change your face. Your face should be good enough and if it isn't, it's other people's problem. And yet I've been part of the theatre industry where it's more critical than any other and where supposedly creative people can't even see beyond what other people look like.

Nevertheless, at age 35, I decided to have the surgery. In a seven-hour operation, the surgical and orthodontic team moved both my lower jaw and my upper mandible further up into my face so that what had been recessed now came forward. The recovery was horrendous; I was off work for two months.

After that operation, eating was a real challenge; I lost quite a few pounds. Luckily I had learned about nutrition and healthy diet. And though I hate exercise, I really worked hard at preparing for surgery. It's a good thing I did, because the aftermath was awful. Whenever I hear people talk about a nip or a tuck, I wonder why anyone would want to go through surgery for strictly cosmetic reasons. It took almost a year for my face to heal and another year for it to settle.

I can see from photographs how different my face really is now. Ironically, the main reason for the surgery—my acting career—no longer exists. I have changed my life focus from theatre to special education for dyslexic children and young adults. Nevertheless, the surgery helped open me to making ongoing changes in my life.

My own dyslexia was never diagnosed when I was growing up. I figured it out myself a couple of years ago when I was reading about the symptoms. It runs in our family; several nieces and nephews have it. That's why I'm so interested in the education of dyslexic children. I have learned so much from my own experience, especially in the arts, about how dyslexics learn successfully; I want to pass it on to others before they get too frustrated and give up on learning and all its possibilities.

On a bad day, my mental image of myself will always be 160 pounds of quirky character actress. I don't think I can ever totally separate my feelings about my personality from those about my appearance. I had gone into the arts and theater because my personality and looks were unusual (I had a big mouth and a big persona), and those two fields didn't require me to be normal-looking or normal-acting. It made a big difference in my life to be considered artistic, especially during the painful and turbulent teen years. I was lucky to find my place in the arty crowd.

I think at some level we always stay at whatever age was critical to our development. It's necessary to like that person, but I wouldn't want to be that teenager again and be as inexperienced as I was then. I felt high school was all foufanetta! In my eyes prom was political! High heels were a sign of oppression!

POSTSCRIPT: By the time I graduated from college, in June of 2000, with my long-sought-after bachelor's degree, my hair had taken on additional meaning and symbolism. It had come to represent not only my quest for an education to help other learning disabled children but also a fitting gift of fitting-in for children with cancer who had lost their hair to chemotherapy. For a full year, I let my hair grow and the week before graduation I donated an eleven-inch braid of my hair to the Locks of Love organization which provides wigs to young cancer patients who want to normalize their appearance. I felt it was the least I could do to help a child who was struggling to fit in, as I had done.

M A R I E, 56:
college professor

I have two memories of my childhood appearance that come from photographs. One positive memory is from the tender age of 1 year, but what I loved about that particular picture was a piece of jewelry that I wore around my neck—two elephants on a chain. The clasp was actually one elephant looped over the other. I loved animals, and this very unique necklace was mine, mine alone. It wasn't my sister's, or handed down to me. I was given this necklace to wear for the picture, taken at our annual sitting with a professional photographer. Between my two sisters, I am gleefully wearing my elephant jewelry. This is one of my very earliest memories, and obviously, I like it very much.

A negative memory is of a coat that I wore to school on the very first day. I started first grade when I was 5, since we didn't have kindergarten in my small town. I wore a hand-me-down brown tweed coat. Some of the buttons had been lost so my mother substituted buttons that didn't exactly match. This was duly recorded on film. Although I did not actually remember wearing this coat, the photograph reminded me.

Even as a young child, I hated my very fine hair. I was bald until I was 2. And finally, when I did get hair, it came out like something my father called "gufa-feathers." It was very fine, blonde hair like a lot of Swedes have. And I continued to have very fine, blonde hair until I was in about fifth grade. Of course, a friend of mine had long, blonde hair in thick braids. It bothered me immensely, this wimpy little hair, which contributed to my negative self-esteem until I developed heavier brown hair.

In a family of tall, thin people, I grew up as the heaviest of all three daughters and my mother and father. I had very large bones and was very muscular. My mother insisted, "Oh dear, you're not fat, you are just husky." And my father lovingly called me "pumpkin" because of my very round face and cheeks. Picking up on this, my sisters called me "pumpkinhead." That contributed nicely to my negative self-image!

I was always large—not fat, but larger than most of the kids in my class. In fact, I grew to my full adult height when I was in eighth grade. I was much taller than any of the boys in my class, but there were several girls my size. That helped a little bit as far as the competition was concerned.

In my teenage years, I actually lived in two worlds, a real world and a fantasy world. In my real world I was husky but smart, competitive and a good student. In my fantasy world I was slim, pretty, and extremely popular with a large crowd of both boyfriends and girlfriends.

When I was 9, 10, and 11, I had a grown-up doll, a pre-Barbie. Because we couldn't buy ready-made doll clothes, we made our own. Even when I was too small to sit down and work the treadle on the sewing machine, Mother allowed me to stand and pedal to sew doll clothes. She had a drawer in the dining room sideboard filled with scraps of fabric, lace pieces, ric rac, and old buttons. I could really fantasize about doll clothes. Out of that drawer I created marvelous costumes. My doll had a bikini, a picture hat, and a portable radio to take to the beach. A wedding dress. Shorts. She was the best-dressed doll in the county and she became my alter ego, in a way. This pastime started my interest in designing and my love of fabrics. My mother never worried about my playing on the sewing machine, and I never sewed over my finger! If I made a mistake, she would pull some stitches for me, but she generally allowed me to make what I wanted. I still have the entire wardrobe for this little doll.

My fantasy world brought me through the cocoon stage of adolescence and helped me a great deal. However, in my junior year in high school, one particular incident really threw me. Each year the seniors willed things to the juniors. I was willed one very thin girl's twenty-four-inch waist! Now, this upset me. It was very cruel. My waist was only about twenty-seven inches but somebody thought this would be very funny. Well, this poor girl herself was so embarrassed, she apologized profusely.

I remember that incident to this day. I cried and cried and ran into the bathroom. Hid out for half a day! That was really the most trying time of my life, the teenage years.

Between my sophomore and junior year in college, I went to work in Yellowstone Park as a waitress. That summer I ate half of what I served and gained thirty pounds. So when I transferred to a new school in September, none of my clothes fit. I had to make myself two quick dresses to start at the new school. I spent most of my early young adult life thinking about losing weight. But as I became more involved in my professional life, started teaching, and became very active in athletics, the weight just naturally came off over a period of years. I was swimming, canoeing, skating, skiing, always doing something. Luckily I wasn't preoccupied with my weight; I just became so involved with other things that appearance took a back seat. And it came out all right. I developed the social and physical me more than the self-interested me. After a couple of years, my weight was more normal, and since then I haven't had much of a problem.

I have always enjoyed textiles and clothing, but originally I started out as an undergraduate in science. I was a very good science student and wanted to go into an applied health field such as medical technology. My mother wanted me to be a nurse, "a good profession for women." The summer between my freshman and sophomore year, I worked in a hospital as a nurses aide to see if this was really for me. I found out I hated hospitals. A nurse simply had to follow directions; there were prescribed things she could do and that was it. Otherwise, call the doctor. And the medical technologist was the most hated person in the hospital, drawing blood from everybody. Also, having spent an entire year ruining my clothes in zoology and chemistry labs, I decided I did not want to spend the rest of my life looking through a microscope at feces, urine, or blood cells! So I cancelled all my science classes and changed my major to my other love, home economics. The physics, chemistry, biology, and physiology were all good background for textiles and foods, so I hadn't wasted my time in those science classes.

During my first years of teaching, I had two very special friends who helped my self-development. One was an English teacher and one was a physical education teacher. They broadened my horizons and introduced me to other worlds: opera, theater, sports, and travel. I became a much more broadly educated and cultured individual. It was through them that I developed a lot of interests and became something more than a home economics teacher. And their friendship really reinforced my feeling of self-worth. I still continue with many of the interests I developed as a young adult, specifically with these two friends.

The other person in my life who truly influences my self-image is my husband. He's my best cheerleader, because he always reinforces what I already like to do and always comments positively on how I look. Thank goodness we agree on aesthetics. I think that if you feel truly loved, then your self-image is improved. He has never been critical, and that has helped a great deal. So these two special friends and my husband have been most important to me in terms of strong self-image.

I see myself in a more positive light these days. I am more accepting of myself, and certainly less concerned about how I am perceived by others. Once I regained my normal weight in college and got beyond young adulthood, I really felt much more desirable. Now I am much more concerned about health than appearance, because when you feel good you look better! A major change in my life is more acceptance of myself. Some time in my mid-30s I became much more positive about myself, after living with my two friends, and then getting married.

I think that my intellect, personality, and achievements outrank my looks. And these things are more important to me. I believe that my self-image is probably higher than the mirror image. I continually forget my age. But I am reminded of it when I look in the mirror, because I see the wrinkles and the grey hair and they sometimes surprise me!

How do I think others perceive me? Some people have commented that I am sophisticated; others have commented on my style. At the end of a weeklong convention, a woman commented that she had noticed what I had worn every day, and thought I had a very interesting style. Students have also commented on this. So what I hope to project, what I do project, and what others perceive seems to be quite consistent.

Others often perceive me as rather stern, and sometimes crabby or no-nonsense. Supposedly, a no-nonsense demeanor is a Scandinavian characteristic, but I think it's more a matter of your upbringing. I am perceived more like my father, who was my role model in life. My sisters are perceived more like my mother, who was always very ladylike.

I think, too, that very often the deportment expected of children during their upbringing is more an issue of class than of nationality. Very often middle-class children were expected to be much more serious and responsible than either lower-class or upper-class children. One of our neighbor families was what we used to call poor, but of the same nationality as our family. They allowed their children to be childlike and to play all the time. They had a box filled with high heels and dresses plus draperies and curtains and stuff. We all loved being queens and kings, dressing up and pretending as much as we liked. We didn't do that sort of thing at home, partially because we were supposed to be more responsible. We were allowed to play, but there was always the expectation that we would be responsible. So my perceived sternness is often just my sense of responsibility.

I am happy with the way I am today, though I'd like to change certain parts of my body that are aging faster than others. Usually I just cover them up so the rest of the world doesn't have to experience the same shock I do! In general, though, I am happy.

How do I plan to deal with the aging process? I plan to stay healthy and to try to keep in shape physically, and to keep company with younger people! I don't want to associate with people my own age who sit and commiserate about getting old. I need to have friends of all different ages. And I plan to continue to be productive and look to the future. This certainly helps in aging gracefully. Taking vitamins helps a great deal, too!

Marsha, 48:
social researcher

My first memory of my appearance as a child was in kindergarten. I compared myself unfavorably with the one perfect little girl in our class. And I came out of that encounter scarred for life! She had gloriously wavy, long, dark auburn hair. I had short, straight, brown hair. She had ringlets. I had cowlicks. Her hair was manageable. My hair stubbornly refused to obey me, my mother, or the neighborhood beautician. Miss Perfect had nonstop dimples. I had a small cleft in my chin, complete with a scar left by the neighbors' porch swing. She had straight, white teeth and a beautiful smile. I had a tentative, gap-toothed smile with saw-edged teeth in a not-so-white color. She had big brown eyes and dark lashes. I had olive eyes with lashes that paled at the ends. Her dresses were starched and immaculate; her shoes were polished. My sash always came untied; my dress was always wrinkled; my shoes were scuffed. She was a Shirley Temple stand-in. I was waif-like long before it became a '90s fashion trend. She was Yin. I was Yang. I never felt I measured up, and I never got over it. Even though I was just like all the rest of the kids in that kindergarten class, I became a 5-year-old aspiring perfectionist. I see it all very clearly now when I look at that kindergarten class photo.

My personal experience of appearance and self-esteem has been under siege for much of my life and has been like a bobsled event. Out of control and whipsawing around, it was initially very negative. When I got some momentum and thought I finally had it under control, it looped back on itself and I had to deal with the same issues from my teenage years all over again. And then just when I thought I was doing fine, I found myself experiencing midlife mechanical breakdowns!

An only child, I was supposed to be a boy—a junior. Unprepared for a girl, my parents named me for my father anyway, using a female variation on Dad's name. The family photographs and stories attest to my uneven progress. I was a scrawny, colicky, 4 1/2-pound preemie with a full head of black hair but doubtful survival skills. Despite all bets to the contrary, I slowly gained weight and blossomed into a charmingly wistful toddler. Once I outgrew my toddler cheekiness, however, I reverted to being a scrawny kid with knobby knees, chapped lips, and cowlicks.

Unpromising in appearance, I was also a sickly child: chronic bronchitis and anemia, extreme cases of measles and chickenpox, ruptured appendix and infected tonsils, mononucleosis, and hemorrhaging from seemingly small injuries. At age 2 I accidentally burned my eyes on a household antibacterial lamp and, for various reasons, my eyes would prove to be a major health and appearance issue for the rest of my life. I was also labeled a picky eater. And klutzy. Spilled my milk at most meals. Ran into things. Forgot to duck other things. I was not exactly prissy, not exactly a tomboy; not exactly graceful, not exactly athletic. I was introverted, shy, and overly sensitive.

Adventuresome or athletic, I was not. Nor was I encouraged to be, beyond the usual girl things. I ice-skated unsteadily, roller-skated well enough, excelled at double-Dutch jump rope, and rode my bike all over the neighborhood. I taught myself to run like a boy because the boys made fun of anyone who ran like a girl. Swimming was my best sport. Esther Williams was my favorite movie star and role model. I was a fish in the water, teaching myself the strokes and tricks that I had seen her do in the movies. However, I never swam competitively or joined a synchronized swimming group.

There was a definite culture of appearance in our family, which affected me positively and negatively. My dad was quite handsome and my mother was stylish and glamorous; they both took pride in their looks and style and often commented negatively on others' shortcomings. Their comments were probably meant to be just humorous or perhaps gossipy, but I picked up on the fact that appearance could easily be disparaged.

My father often told a story about his bachelor days: He and a friend were driving through town when they spotted two young women walking along the sidewalk ahead of them. Appreciative of the women's figures from the back, the men whistled. When one of the women turned around, revealing facial features that apparently didn't meet expectations, my father called out to her, "Not you, dogface!" This story still haunts me, because, although I never thought of my father as unkind, the intended humor of this story is devastatingly cruel. The lesson was not lost on me—an extremely shy, overly sensitive, unpretty little girl. The world could be unmerciful to those who didn't measure up to the standard, whatever the standard was.

As a child, I heard my parents describe me as excruciatingly shy, skinny, and knobby-kneed, with untameable hair. I don't remember that they ever said I was pretty or pleasing or personable while I was growing up. The popular admonition, "If you can't say something nice, then don't say anything at all," made me feel that if my parents never affirmed my appearance, it must not measure up. Then, too, one of my mother's favorite expressions was, "She's so homely she's cute!" and, although she never said it directly to me, I came to feel the comment applied to me.

I was raised as "Mommy's girl," expected to be "seen and not heard," well-behaved at all times, and to reflect well on my mother's child-rearing practices—all pretty typical stuff for girls of my era. My father was, as they say, undemonstrative. I didn't have much of a relationship with him or get much positive attention from him. Most often he reminded me to walk with my head up because, being both nearsighted and shy, I had a habit of looking down all the time. Often, too, he reminded me to smile.

I realize now that I didn't smile much because my mother didn't. She disliked the gaps and spaces in her teeth. When she laughed, she covered her mouth with her hand. She always said she didn't like her long nose, her long neck or her short legs. She was, in fact, slim and well-proportioned. Very aware of appearance and style, she played up her resemblance to Joan Crawford. She was creatively talented, designing and making many of her own clothes in the movie star mode. Wrapping herself in glamour, she enhanced what she saw as her physical shortcomings. My mother was admittedly insecure about her looks and background and used bravado of personality and body language to compensate. Unfortunately, she made me her confidante in all these matters. She talked, I listened. Unfortunately, I took it personally and integrated it all into my own sense of self, as kids do. What I learned about self-confidence from her was mostly camouflage in the form of clothes, accessories and body language. By the time that kindergarten photo was taken, I was already convinced that I needed a lot of work in terms of looks and personality.

Both my parents were avid golfers, and that fact, along with Dad's health, motivated our nomadic lifestyle. My dad organized his business to allow extended trips to the South during the winter months. So from the third grade through the eighth grade, I started each school year in September in my midwestern hometown, transferring to a second school in Florida at Thanksgiving. Then, sometime after Easter, I left the school in Florida, returning to my hometown for the remainder of the school year. This unusual arrangement always produced a galloping case of throw-ups in me during the first week of school in Florida, following every one of those yearly transfers. It caused me to have to play academic catch-up in Florida and to feel very socially insecure in both schools. I never felt as if I belonged at either school, but my sense of isolation was worse in the hometown school with my two short sessions of attendance separated by both the winter absence and the summer vacation. Needless to say, my innate introversion was heightened by this social and academic hopscotching.

To complicate matters, my shaky self-image took a severe nosedive at age 9 when I acquired very thick glasses for acute nearsightedness. My delight at being able to see so much better with my new glasses soon disappeared with the advent of another of Mother's sayings. "Boys don't make passes at girls who wear glasses!" Now I was not only quiet, plain, bookish, insecure and a transient, but I also had thick ugly glasses. I smiled even less. Already a golf orphan, I became a real loner, spending most of my time reading, sewing, watching television, and introverting.

However, I loved to play dress-up in Mom's glamorous clothes and to make doll clothes. Inspired by my mother's creative handwork, I began making clothes for my Toni doll. From there I graduated to making my own clothes. First experiments aside, I slowly developed my own talent and fashion sense. Although, during the teen years, I blossomed creatively at the sewing machine, at the same time I hid behind it socially. My creativity was intensified by my isolation and limited social life. My fantasies of glamour, inspired by the movies, took flight with fabrics and patterns. One of my friends jokes that Catholic school uniforms prevented her from ever learning how to dress herself; I insist that Catholic school uniforms fueled my obsession with clothes. Eventually I achieved a certain aura of small-town celebrity due to my creative endeavors and was continually urged by friends to do something with my talent.

By age 9 I was experiencing the prelude to all my hormonal changes. By the age of 11 I had matured physically and was experiencing the mood swings and painful side effects of my newly acquired femininity. A month-long bout of menstrual hemorrhaging put me in the hospital for a D & C and gave me grave doubts about this growing-up stuff! Like many young girls, I was very put off by the intensity of bodily changes: long, painful, and erratic menses; excessive nervous perspiration; oily skin; too much dark body hair; recalcitrant acne; seborrheic dandruff; and painful fears of social isolation.

I began to see my body as the enemy and continued to do so for years. It continually conspired against me, making me feel helpless and frustrated. My pursuit of perfectionism was frustrated to the nth degree. During high school years my best friend's favorite expression, "For a fat girl who sweats a lot you sure don't smell bad!" always hit too close to home for my sweat-stained comfort! It seems there was an insensitive expression that matched each of my many sensitivities!

If I was shy and introverted in general, I was painfully uncomfortable around boys. Although some of my grade school classmates had started dating in fifth grade, my first experiences with house parties and school dances were dreadful. I would have been happier at home with a book. Ages 11, 12, and 13 were painful and lonely. By the time I was in seventh grade, we had moved into a new suburban neighborhood in my hometown where my sense of isolation was pretty much complete and my self-image was shaky. I commuted back to the old neighborhood for seventh and eighth grade but spent two lonely summers in the new house before entering high school.

My freshman yearbook photo, in which I have a severe expression, basic ponytail, acne and thick glasses, is pretty grim. However, staying in one school made it easier to make friends and, in an all-girls Catholic school, I didn't have to worry about dealing with boys—at least for the time being. My lifelong friend Colleen and I met in homeroom on the first day of high school. Personality-wise she was everything I wasn't: bright, funny, outgoing, and light-hearted! And so again I found someone to compare myself with, self-defeatingly, for many years. Only now it was my personality that suffered from my own unfair comparisons. When my dad commented on how delightful Colleen was, I figured he liked her better than me.

At the beginning of my sophomore year and at my mother's instigation, I acquired contact lenses along with a permed "poodle" hairstyle. This was the first major transformation of my appearance. Slowly I began to acquire an outward sophistication born of travel, reading, and television that hid my social naiveté, an intellectual ability that hid my inexperience, and a facade of self-possession that hid reticence and insecurity. At age 15, my early maturation and serious demeanor often caused me to be mistaken for an 18-year-old. However, my chronic acne, which even X-ray treatments couldn't quell, still caused me great frustration and kept my potential spontaneity locked behind my self-consciousness.

I was always a good student, well-behaved, mild-mannered, and overly conscientious. I was consistently on the honor roll. As a result, any frustrations or problems I had in school or in my social life were pretty much dismissed as unimportant by my mother, who also counseled that girls were wise to obfuscate an overabundance of intelligence. "No nice young men will want to take you out on dates, or marry you, if you are too smart!" When, in my sophomore year of high school, the teachers automatically steered me into the college prep elective courses for the next two years, my father failed to see the point. Why did I, a girl, need to go to college? "Just take typing and shorthand and plan to be a secretary, like your mother was, until you get married!"

This was not an unusual attitude among the large local Catholic families, but because I was an only child and academically inclined, it hadn't occurred to me that I wouldn't be encouraged to go to college. My cousin Marianne was attending college on scholarship; my mother had spoken of her endeavor appreciatively, I thought. Apparently, it had never occurred to my father and mother that I would want to continue on with school and they had given no thought to issues of college tuition or the fact that although my grades might qualify me for a scholarship, my father's income would disqualify me. Somehow, after some mood storms and some discussion, the issue was resolved in my favor. Along with Latin, I took chemistry and physics and graduated from high school as a member of the National Honor Society, in spite of my mother's admonitions!

This incident looms large in my life. I subsequently developed a great deal of ambivalence about college, career goals and motivations, which didn't become clear to me until many years later. This ambivalence caused me to back off many potential goals, and start zigzagging through life.

Unable to identify a major that really interested me, I dropped out of the college I had argued to attend, and enrolled in a fashion design school in New York. But then I didn't think I was talented enough to pursue the career in fashion design to which I had aspired. Although these defaulted decisions have caused me much self-doubt and many recriminations, I have recently reevaluated these harsh self-judgments in a more positive light. But for years my ambivalence and lack of self-confidence caused me much disappointment.

In the years since my first physical transformation as a high school sophomore, I have experimented with my appearance with varying results. Two years in New York and a six-week trip to Europe with Colleen gave me several new layers of confidence. I was more outgoing, more at ease, more personable, and sardonically humorous. I actually liked the way I looked at that point, although my stubborn acne still kept me frustrated and self-conscious until about age 25 when I finally found a way to get it under control with medication.

In spring of 1967 I moved to Chicago, where I soon met my future husband. He once said he was initially drawn to me because I was attractive and smart and well-dressed, a combination the likes of which he had not encountered in college or graduate school. This statement flew in the face of all my mother's admonitions! How could I resist? I was attracted to him because he was nice-looking, sincere, smart, ambitious and wearing a camelhair overcoat with epaulets, the likes of which I had not encountered on other Chicagoans of the male species. They all wore ratty tan trench coats! How could I resist?

In 1971, as a young married woman, I returned to college to complete my degree requirements. Pleased to have accomplished that goal, I was still pretty unfocused on what exactly to do with my life. But I had my sheepskin in hand at last.

During my 20s—as a single, engaged and newly married young woman—I felt very attractive; however, my comfort level with myself was cut short soon enough. I developed a severe case of chronic corneal erosion in my right eye. (The outer layers of corneal tissue slough off spontaneously, leaving a raw spot on the surface of the eye until the cornea can regenerate itself.) Incredibly painful, each occurrence initially required large pressure bandages on the eye for a week or more at a time, along with drops and enforced inactivity. The corneal erosion precluded any further use of my contact lenses and necessitated a return to the thick ugly glasses, often worn balanced on the end of my nose over the dreaded pressure bandages. My hard-won self-image plummeted!

While I worked in the corporate world, the glasses probably gave me a more serious demeanor (as if I really needed one!) in a rather chauvinistic environment. However, I felt unattractive all over again and hid myself and my personality behind my glasses. With the return of my ugly glasses and the sudden resurgence of my teenage acne, I went back to seeing myself as that introverted, plain, unsmiling, "blemished" and serious person I had been as a high school freshman. And although my experience of the corporate world was often frustrating, it did provide the opportunity for much personal growth and increased self-confidence. Something was working in my favor.

The acne was re-attacked and re-conquered with several years worth of strong medication. The corneal erosion problem lasted about 15 years, tapering off in severity but often requiring eye drops, unguents, and rest, if not bandages. In addition, my extreme nearsightedness had put me in jeopardy for detached retinas with potential for vision loss. While contact lenses had provided some protection from further vision deterioration, glasses were known to actually encourage increased nearsightedness. And bifocals were now an imminent necessity!

In 1989 I was referred to an ophthalmologist who specialized in radial keratotomy, a surgical procedure which could dramatically correct nearsightedness and reduce the threat of detached retinas. The doctor said he could dramatically improve my vision, eliminate the need for bifocals, and hold off the retinal problems.

All this was promised in a simple operation. The two separate surgeries—right eye and left eye, six weeks apart—went well enough, but the complications from corneal erosion caused the most excruciatingly painful experience of my life. Each operation required an extended recuperation period of four days in bed in a darkened room wearing pressure bandages and using codeine painkillers, that, excuse the expression, "barely scratched the surface!"

Once my corneas healed and I no longer needed glasses, the image transformation was quite spectacular. When my face came out from behind my glasses, my personality and sense of humor reemerged, my smile increased by kilowatts, and much of my old self-consciousness faded. I felt like a brand new butterfly! And I finally began to see myself and experience myself as attractive, accomplished, intelligent, credible, personable, and funny. I looked better than ever at that point in my life and certainly felt better than ever about myself, despite the fact that I had just learned I had discernible cataracts.

When I left the corporate world in early 1988, I started a small business as an image consultant for professional women and became deeply involved in the psychology of appearances. My seemingly erratic career path was now heading towards an identifiable goal. The several aspects of fashion design, image consulting, the psychology of appearances, and interviewing women about their appearance issues has come together in a meaningful way as my life's interest—even if it has taken a long time to coalesce.

The experience of being female has never been easy or comfortable for me. Various physical problems and strong undercurrents of moodiness, along with a generally pessimistic outlook on life have made it hard for me to truly "enjoy being a girl" or to feel in control of my body. With age and experience have come more acceptance, comfort and ease with myself and with life, but I have no illusions that it will ever be easy for me to look consistently on the bright side. On a good day my dark viewpoint is integral to my dark sense of humor; on a bad day it can be a downer!

I don't remember getting much positive feedback about my physical appearance or personality through the tough growing-up years. Or perhaps I just couldn't hear it. In the absence of affirmation, I usually assumed the worst about myself. It has only been during the past six years (post-glasses II) that I have been able to receive and hear the positive feedback about my looks, my personality, and my abilities from the vantage point of a new perspective.

During those long years behind my glasses, I had taken up skiing, sailing, tennis, and scuba diving. The transition to a more athletic lifestyle has given me more competence, confidence, body awareness, and fitness than ever before. I like being a jock who cleans up well into a glamorous female.

Fortunately, feminism, age, and renewed spirituality have begun to neutralize the effect of the cultural stereotypes of appearance and personality, which, in my youth, gripped me so tenaciously. My appearance is congenial to me now. I feel that I am attractive, somewhat unconventional looking, with good bone structure. I am pleased that I now know the most flattering hairstyles and makeup techniques for my features. It only took me 48 years to like what I see in the mirror!

Fortunately, too, I have been able to redesign my self-image and redefine myself and my goals. My personality is still unconventional though very different from my youthful one. I would say that my whole package of ability, achievement, personality, and looks are in pretty good shape and well enough balanced these days. I am okay with who I am, even if I'm not perfect. I have some new educational goals to pursue and I intend to stay physically active and intellectually probing as long as possible.

POSTSCRIPT #1: Just when I felt more together and in control of my life than ever before, I was diagnosed with breast cancer. At age 51, my prime time, it was a real shock. Is it the Marines who say, "What doesn't kill you makes you stronger"? It's true. The bad news was cancer; the good news was catching it early! I was so busy trying to find a way to end-around menopause I hadn't even considered the possibility of cancer.

Until the day I learned of my malignancy, I viewed aging as a matter of staying fit and locating appropriate role models to emulate. I thought I had it made. The experience seemed terrifyingly surreal and yet some very wonderful things came out of it: friendship, affection, love and concern. Illness took away my sense of control and yet it returned much human warmth and caring. My family and friends have made me feel truly treasured. Still, if I fear anything about aging, it is ill health of the debilitating kind. Even with so many loving friends I will surely need to develop a large reservoir of patience and insight to deal with this aging business.

POSTSCRIPT #2: At age 54, my vision is now markedly diminishing again due to cataracts. Surgery and a return to glasses are inevitable, but so are new visions—travel, publication—and new challenges—graduate school, golf and perhaps even optimism!

The past several years have given me a chance to rethink a lot of things, to ask myself questions, and to search for answers. The second half of a woman's life is supposed to be exciting, fulfilling, challenging and blossoming with new potential and goals. Much of the first half of my life felt punishing; I hope to live the second half as an adventure and thereby enjoy the scenery, the ride, and the experiences.

M A R Y, 48:
primary school teacher

A photograph triggers one of my first memories of my appearance. It shows me with a snowman I had made. I am wearing a coat my mother had fashioned of someone else's coat. Although my parents were really frugal and wouldn't buy a new coat for me, this was the cutest little plaid coat. It was a pretty shade of blue with brightly colored lines running through it. And it had a cute little hat with it. I remember liking the coat except that the fabric was scratchy; I didn't like that too much.

Some of the negative things about myself had to do with wearing that same darn coat as I tried to learn to ride a tricycle. I couldn't get my legs to work the pedals to make the stupid thing go. And I couldn't steer it, either. I would get over to the edge of the sidewalk, get my little wheels stuck, and then fall over on my side. I hated that even more than the stupid tricycle. Even when my dad put blocks on the pedals so I could reach them better, I still couldn't steer it. I guess I couldn't figure out how to push on the pedals and steer the handlebars at the same time. I finally solved that problem, but I didn't ride a two-wheeler until I was in first grade. I wasn't really coordinated.

But I always thought I was cute! My mother made sausage curls with my hair, spending a lot of time with it; she used to tell me how shiny my hair was and how she loved the natural curls and waves. She made those curls by winding them around her finger and brushing them so they would all fall just perfectly. And she bought me little wide-brimmed straw hats to show off the curls. I always had patent leather shoes for Easter. We Catholics laugh about black patent leather shoes but they were a must.

I was a shy child and I felt bad about that. My parents were very protective of us children and I had a strong sense of Mom and Dad and family. I wasn't shy in my family, but strangers really scared me. In today's world it would probably be a good thing, but in those days it was a negative. I was very shy until I got to know people and then I yackety-yacked. I hung out with and yacked to the neighbor ladies, who were wonderful.

As far as physical characteristics go, I sucked my thumb for the longest time and I was always embarrassed about needing that oral gratification. Luckily it didn't do anything to my teeth. They protrude a little bit in front but not much.

I don't remember much positive reinforcement from my brother, David, who is four and a half years older than I am. I think he was probably jealous of me. Mom read stories to us and we played together, but I don't remember ever feeling anything special about him—not even that he was my big brother and I wanted to tag around with him. It wasn't until later that I found out he felt protective of me. In second grade one of the neighborhood boys came up behind me, tackled me, threw me on the ground, and started beating up on me. Suddenly my brother came roaring out of the house, grabbed that kid by the neck, and threw him into the neighbor's yard. Otherwise, David just teased me constantly. I hated that.

My dad wasn't around much; he worked very odd hours doing shift work. But when I got a little older I was more of a boy to him than my brother was. While David went off and did things with his own buddies, Dad and I would go fishing and hunting.

My friends and schoolmates affected me both positively and negatively. When I was in second grade, I had a good friend, also named Mary. During that year the nuns led Mary and me to believe that, as the two shortest girls in the class, both of us would lead the first Holy Communion procession. Well, in the late spring of that year, we had the May crowning ceremony, in which we were to wear our pretty white dresses. But as it turned out, the one and only leader on this occasion would be the shortest girl. I wanted that honor so badly, but I swear that Mary, my friend, bent her knees so she could be the shortest one. I remember lining up along the blackboard chalk troughs while fighting with her about who was the shortest one. Mary must have crouched so she was the shortest, because I think I was really shorter.

When I was in eighth grade, my dad broke both his legs in an awful accident in the mill where he worked. Then the company owners claimed that he couldn't keep up as well as before, and suggested that he take retirement or leave the company. They offered to match whatever he had in the retirement fund as severance pay, but the amount was practically nothing for a man in his early 40s with a wife and four children. So for years he travelled 80 miles to work at another job. Mom didn't want to move away from her family, so he commuted, living there during the week and driving back and forth every weekend during all my high school years. It was awful.

Throughout my high school years, I always felt as if I was playing catch-up with everybody else. I wanted to be with the group from the east side because I knew Marsha and Ellie. But I always felt a little behind every-body—a little more innocent. Maybe the rest of that group was fairly innocent, but later on when Ellie and Diane used to talk so freely about what they did with the guys it floored me. So I just always felt that I couldn't keep up with the group I wanted to be with. And I probably threw myself into some things that I shouldn't have, dating wild guys and juvenile delinquent types. However, when my mom would give me the "look" in regard to my social circle, I wasn't going to go against her and keep seeing those guys.

I used to come in late and make all kinds of excuses—the stuff that we all did—but I would never hurt my mom. She usually made sensible rules but even if she laid down the law it was okay. Of course, I pushed right up to the edge like everybody else, but knowing she had all the responsibility for us during the week when my dad was gone, I didn't really cause trouble.

In grade school, my friend Marcie had a special way of making me feel good about myself by sharing secrets and doing fun things. Mark, one of my first loves, did wonderful things for my self-image during sixth, seventh, and eighth grades. A boy named John did, too; we liked each other a lot in grade school. He was good-looking, one of the studs in the class, you might say. And since he liked me that made me feel good about myself.

Then for a while I dated a guy named Mike, who was quite a bit older and a real cutie; he was from the east side of town and had a car. I snuck out sometimes to ride around in the car with him. I did those kinds of things and I also started smoking with my friend Rosie, who was always so much more grown up than anybody.

It wasn't really until college that I felt truly shot down. There were very few of us newly admitted coeds on the local college campus in those days. Although the fraternities were always picking a homecoming queen or a military ball queen, they picked the same women every time; I was never chosen. And I was really upset over that because I thought I was pretty good-looking. I remember feeling very discouraged during my four years there. After we started dating, my husband Steve told me that his fraternity had considered running me but it just never came through. I figured I wasn't feminine enough or something. I still can't figure that one out; it put my self-image down a little.

Although I thought I was pretty in high school and college, I couldn't figure out why I never got the attention of the guys I wanted to date. Certainly I went to all those high school mixers at the boys' school, as well as park dances and CYO dances. And all those college mixers, too. And I flirted with everybody, but they didn't get the message, I guess. I must have been "looking for love in all the wrong places." We were kind of boy-crazy in those days!

For a while in college I dated a fellow named Larry who surely helped alleviate those worrisome feelings. I have always liked guys, and I realize now that I related to guys much better than to girls. Maybe my relationship with my dad promoted that. I usually liked the things that guys talked about.

So dating Larry for a while and then dating and marrying Steve were positive experiences for me. Steve was great; he made me feel good about myself. He always had a very cutting wit that I admired, and although he's short, he was more than just cute: he was extremely strong and tough-looking. As a football player, he was short but physically well-developed. And in those college days it was the crewcut and those gorgeous eyes—those twinkly black eyes. My kind of stuff.

But how about this for a world-class put-down? Steve graduated a year ahead of me, and when I was a senior in college, he decided that he might have a vocation to the priesthood. So he called me long-distance from graduate school to say he was going to pursue this idea. I said, "Well, does this mean that our relationship is over?" When he said, "Yes, I think it better be over," I was upset and really taken aback. I hung up the phone and just stood there. I had no idea that he was even thinking this stuff. I couldn't believe the guy. And then he got drunk a few nights later and called and said, "Forget about the priesthood thing!"

I told him to call back when he was sober and serious, and to have Father O'Brien, our friend over at the college, call me if this was for real. So when Father O'Brien called to say we needed a little counseling, I said, "Yes, I think we do!" It was several months before we decided that we would take up where we left off. That was my young adulthood. There wasn't much time between college and marriage. We did do a formal engagement ceremony, which was very lovely and solemn, in the chapel at the college. We didn't have engagement rings, but we signed a document to pledge our troth.

We were married in November after Steve came back from army officers basic training. We were supposed to be stationed in Hawaii, but when we got there the army said, "Don't unpack; you are going to Vietnam." We had only been married six weeks when Steve left. I came back home but eventually returned to Hawaii to establish residency and wait for Steve to return. My young adulthood was obviously pretty chaotic and disorganized for a while. We came home, settled in a small town, and raised our two boys. And life has flowed along fairly smoothly for our family. There were no major catastrophes—just the day-to-day kids, pets, sports, work, school, PTA, mom and dad stuff. Just being on top of all that made me feel good about myself.

I know that people have always perceived me as cute; even now they see me that way because I am small. Some years ago I was working in the local public library adjacent to City Hall. A fellow who worked in City Hall and came over to the library regularly always patted me on the head in passing. It bothers me enough that I'm short, but to be patted on the head as an adult in my 30s was too much. So I have trouble with being cute. Here I am closing in on 50 and people still see me as cute. I would prefer vivacious, although I don't mind pretty. Vivacious is really how I describe myself, and that's what I think I am. I have some lingering shyness and lack of self-assurance that I still feel, so I see myself as vulnerable but also as bouncy and outgoing.

Sometimes people perceive me as a little bit scattered. Now that I am teaching grammar school again, I think perhaps my students perceive me as somewhat flaky because they are often quite protective of me. I perceive myself as wanting to be protected, but why my young students feel so protective of me, I don't know.

Kids tend to see an adult as in control, organized, efficient and directed. When my students get to know me, they say, "'Mrs. Mayhem' is just not like that!" I tell them in class right away that I learn as much from them as they learn from me. I want them to realize that I am also human; there are lots of things that I goof up and forget. So I understand their excuses about forgetting as long as it doesn't happen too often. In that way I try to turn my self-perceived flakiness into an object lesson for my students. That's what it's all about: turning your liabilities into assets as well as a learning experience.

I think that I dress, talk, and act a lot like who I really am; I am pretty together. My looks were best in my 30s, but I don't mind getting older. In my 30s everything came together and I was at the right weight. When I hit 40, things changed but I don't mind some of the aging things. It's more acceptable to age now; it's the baby boomer thing. At one time I wanted to save money for a little plastic surgery, but now I think not; I feel comfortable enough with myself. To me it's not so important to look young as to think young. And that's what I want to keep doing. I hope my image of myself and my personality doesn't age. I don't care about the outside of my body so much, although I do dye my hair.

I know people perceive me as very efficient, organized, and knowledgeable, but I am always floored that people see me as more outgoing, focused, and directed than I think I am. Wow, I am really a good actress!

MAUREEN, 48:
community volunteer

My first memory of my appearance, from age 3 or 4, has to do with fingernail polish. My godmother, Mary, who would come in from out of town and stay overnight with us, always polished my nails because I loved her red nail polish. My mother was plain but my godmother was "fancy" and came from Chicago, which made her fascinating. Mary also had a routine for cleansing her face and putting on her make-up which I loved to sit and watch.

The other thing I remember was that people always commented on how cute my dimple was, so I thought I was really something. I was doted on like a little princess, although the family never used the word princess. We lived in the same building as the family business, a country restaurant and bar. It was a big place filled with people: my widowed grandmother lived with us, and one of the bartenders and one of the waitresses also lived in the building. With a built-in audience of family, employees, and customers, I used to dance a lot with my father. People always complimented me on my dimple and my dancing.

I spent first grade in a country school; everybody was in one room. Then, because my mother wanted my brother and me to go to Catholic school, she organized a bus to take the kids in our area into town to St. Willard's School. My friend Jenny and I rode the school bus together every day until I completed my freshman year of high school. In that country setting I didn't have a lot of peers with whom to compare myself. I was just glad to have one friend; we didn't look at appearances very much when we were growing up.

During that period, dance gave me many positive experiences. I had taken lessons from the time I was 3 years old, so dressing up and performing was a big part of my life. I was good; I had some talent. Dancing continued to give me some status and a lot of confidence throughout high school. When I was a freshman I started teaching dance classes in our home-studio, and running that little business gave me all kinds of publicity, popularity, and pocket money.

From the time my hair was long enough, my grandma and my mother put rag curls in my hair. I didn't like them because I had such thin hair; between each rag curl was four inches of scalp, it seemed. I hated all those spaces on my head and those wimpy little curls hanging down. And my hair really bothered me when I went to visit my cousin Dora, who was the only person I ever compared myself with. She had beautiful, heavy, thick hair and wore the same kind of curls, which were thick and shiny and just perfect. But that was the only negative feeling I had—when I went to visit Dora, because I wasn't as pretty and my hair wasn't as nice as hers. Although my mother said that I had more talent and personality, to me those things didn't count.

A special appearances ritual that I remember while growing up was visiting hat shops. Although my mother had been a seamstress and made all our clothes, she loved to buy hats. For Easter my grandmother, my mother, and I always went shopping for new hats. The three of us would try on hats for hours. That was a big deal all the way through high school.

I didn't always like the clothes my mother made for me. When I started taking the school bus into town, I saw that the city kids didn't have home-made clothes; theirs were store-bought. The one thing that I really coveted was a pair of frontier pants with those pearl button snaps on the pockets. Not only would my mother not buy me a pair, she would not let me wear slacks of any kind, even to a Sunday matinee. She didn't think slacks or pants were appropriate.

Being dressed up and looking nice was very important, especially on Sunday—particularly because we had the kind of business we did, a restaurant-tavern. My mother made a big deal of going to church on Sunday, all dressed up, with our heads held high because our business could be perceived as either negative or positive. In the country, of course, it was positive, a social place where everyone gathered on Sunday. But in town, when kids asked what my parents did, it wasn't so easy to say, "We own a tavern."

Mostly I had positive feelings about myself. I had learned to socialize with adults at a young age because my parents expected me to meet and greet people, to visit with them, and to get along. I learned a lot about being with the public and how to act. My brother took the attitude that it wasn't his job and therefore he never learned to converse with people, but I was put up front as the little showpiece. Mum would tell the customers I was a dancer and then encourage me to start up the record player, put on a costume, and dance. I wasn't a commercial entertainment package *per se*, but everyone in the community knew that I was a dancer.

I didn't have any real traumatic experiences when I started my period in sixth grade, but when my face started breaking out in seventh grade, that really bothered me. I was one of the few kids my age who saw a dermatologist during seventh and eighth grade and who had to use a face-peeling medication. I dealt with that situation by becoming extremely conscious of my hands and nails: keeping my nails filed and polished, wearing rings, drawing attention to my hands rather than my face.

All my life I have hated my high forehead. I grew up with bangs; I didn't know how to avoid them. I tried several different hairstyles in high school, but my real problem was not having enough hair to cover my high forehead. I have had many different styles in my life—long, short, permed, straight, forward, back—because I didn't know what to do. And it was all to hide my forehead.

During my grade school years people began to call me skinny, which really bothered me. Being flat-chested at the same time didn't help. My godmother saw the pain I was going through and always said, "Your personality is more important!" If I hadn't had her to tell me, "We will get through this," it would have been much harder because I compared myself with my cousin Dora, who seemed to be filling out much more.

In the later teenage years, my appearance didn't bother me too much; I didn't really have a lot of negative feelings. My complexion problems were under control. I had learned how to put on makeup for dance recitals and performances and had also learned a lot about everyday makeup. I still wasn't pleased with my thin hair; however, the flip was the popular style, so once my hair grew longer I felt more comfortable.

Extracurricular activities at school always got me into one group or another and gave me a chance to mix and meet people. By the time I got into young adulthood I had some good friends. Dating wasn't a bad experience, either. I went out with lots of fellows who were involved with the musicals we staged in high school and college.

There was, however, one really negative experience connected with dating. Mum had always said that if I looked nice and acted nice, people would accept me. I felt I was as good as anyone else: I was verbal, involved, and a good student. But I got hurt badly when Russ broke up with me. His mother felt I was from the wrong side of the tracks, which was hard to take because I never felt that way. I felt country versus city; and, maybe, lower class versus middle class. But my parents owned a business and that was the way up and out of the working class. Without an education, that's all they could do and I respected that. I knew my grandparents were farmers; I didn't have any qualms about that either. But when Russ said his mother didn't think he should be dating me, it wasn't hard to figure out why. That was devastating!

My friends and I didn't talk much about college until our last year in high school. Not everyone was going to college; we were all trying to decide what to do. I had no encouragement from my parents to go to college; they just wanted me to teach dancing. But when I heard other people talking about college, I wanted to go and that's when I realized I was going to be left behind. A college education was just out of the question financially; I had saved only enough money to go to the local Catholic college for a semester. The second semester I audited because, although I was still teaching dancing, I didn't have enough tuition money. The next semester I decided to quit and go to Europe for a different experience.

I talked my friend Kris into joining me. Surprisingly, my parents didn't fight me on it. It was a real adventure and I had the guts to carry it out; I wasn't afraid. My mother made most of my clothes for the trip, and everything was fine except for the incident involving the red dress.

Kris and I had an appointment for an audience with the Pope; Kris's parish priest, Father Dave, who was attending the North American College in Rome, had helped us with the arrangements. We were to meet him first, in the center of St. Peter's Square, for a tour. He was there waiting for us and as we approached he blushed to high heaven.

Something was obviously wrong, but we couldn't figure out what it was. We knew we couldn't wear slacks for this occasion, and we each had one dress with us for the papal audience. Kris's dress was black and mine was red. Father Dave took one look at me and said, "Did you have to wear red?" I said, "It's the only dress I have. Why?" He simply said, "That's okay," and dropped it. By the time we went to lunch, everybody was making comments in Italian to Father Dave and he was blushing wildly! When I asked him what was going on, he said, "Well, it's your red dress! It's bad enough for a priest to be with two young women. But for one of them to be wearing a red dress is advertising, you know—your profession!" That was how we found out that in Italy only hookers wore red. That was an experience I sure wasn't prepared for.

By the time I finally went back to college, I was married and had two kids. Going to school actually came about because of dancing. I was choreographing the summer theater program staged by the music department of our local Catholic college. At the cast party, I became engrossed in conversation with a German fellow named Peter. When he found out I hadn't finished college, he was appalled. I explained that I didn't have enough money at the time. "Well, why don't you finish now?" he insisted, and I said I couldn't really think of any reason. Peter was relentless. He went so far as to talk to my husband on the side, so later when I brought it up, Jerry said if I could handle it he sure didn't care if I enrolled.

Really scared to go back to college at age 27, I registered for an audited course. I was almost ten years older than everybody else; nobody my age was going back to college in those days. That first class was a huge sociology class with 300 students. I still remember my fear of walking in that first day and sitting in room 006. Everyone else was ready for the lecture to begin, but I didn't know how to put up the stupid lap desk, which was folded down to my right. When I finally wiggled it around and got it over my lap, I was sweating; I thought everybody in that room was watching me. It was one of the few times in my life that I felt lacking in confidence; and it was over such a stupid thing. I almost quit—I felt so dumb.

I got going and really liked sociology 101; but when I got a C on the midterm exam, it did not sit well with me. I literally did not know that because I had been away from school for so long, I had to learn how to learn all over again. I asked the only other adult in the class, a nun, to help me and we studied together for the final exam. That gave me the success and the momentum I needed. With an A for the course, I decided to go back to school full-time and the registrar transferred my grade for credit. The second semester I took three courses as a full-time student.

That was the first time in my life I bought a pair of jeans! Everybody else was wearing jeans in 1970, and my conservative slacks made me look like a grown woman coming back to school. I had to buy jeans to fit in. I had always hated them. I hadn't even been buying them for my own kids to wear to school. But at that point, with my first jeans—hip-huggers, with bell bottoms—I was pretty hot stuff.

I also got a pair of wire-rims because I needed glasses to read the blackboard. I really tried to avoid the middle-class housewife look. Even though I knew a couple of the teachers socially, I tried to fit in with the kids as much as possible and they pretty much accepted me. When one smart-ass kid said, "I suppose you just read *Time* magazine," I didn't even know it was an insult. I realized I had a lot to learn and needed to be a little bit more radical.

Going back to school at that time in my life was about being radical. It was totally different from when I had gone to college for one semester in 1961. Back then, everything was sororities and fraternities and fun. By the early 1970s the school had dropped fraternities and sororities; there were no more homecoming parades. Kids were protesting the Vietnam War. I declared sociology as my major: I liked dealing with wide-ranging issues, and meeting some of the European staff at school just fed my interest. There was another world out there besides hometown, USA.

Once I knew school wasn't all that big a deal, it wasn't such an over-whelming obstacle in my life. When I realized that I was intelligent, capable, and highly motivated, I became apologetic for getting all A's. I heard myself saying, "Well, I'm not as busy as you kids are. I don't have to run here and there." In reality, of course, I was going home to make supper and take care of the kids, and then studying between 10 at night and 2 in the morning. I lived on very little sleep, but I loved the stimulation. I was completely focused. The younger students were not.

I never apologized for going back to school, but I didn't know how to answer when people asked, "What are you going to do when you gradu-ate?" I got so sick of those questions; I finally started saying I was going for the education, period.

As far as I can remember, no one ever told me I was pretty. I had other things going for me and I was encouraged to develop my person-ality. But I don't remember any guys I went out with ever calling me pretty: their flattery came in other forms, "You look nice! You're a good dancer." Yet, through the years, people have come up to me and said, "Gee, your husband is really good-looking," so I guess I've always felt that Jerry was the more attractive of the two of us. Also, now that my daughters, especially Valerie, are older, people often compare us. Very often they say how pretty she is. So if I really need it, I will deduce that I must be pretty and that Valerie got it from Jerry and me! Then, too, I remind my husband how important it is for him to tell me I look nice! Those words are priceless.

Although I don't like letting myself go physically, I have done just that because I don't put myself first: the kids come first, the new washer and dryer comes first. I tell myself I don't need to get a perm or have my hair done. One reason is that I haven't wanted to spend the money—always a big issue in my marriage—on myself because Jerry works on commission and I never know what the budget will look like at the end of the month. Also I have that strong Catholic concept of self-sacrifice: being selfish is wrong and you cannot think of yourself. I've recently decided that idea is self-negating and I've got to balance it. That's one of the things I am working on.

Once in a while, when I see someone who looks good, I realize I could work a little harder and look a little sharper. But, although I looked better when I was younger, I feel better about myself now. I feel together, confident, and competent.

I think most people like me and respect my mind. They ask for my advice. I was invited to join the board of the citywide day care organization a few years ago because they said I was a critical thinker and not afraid to talk. I think that's because I don't care if people disagree with me, although I would like them to see my point. I find debate intellectually stimulating. I get excited about issues and passionate about ideas and causes.

Right now I'm not clear about what my achievement in life has been. I don't think I'm finished yet. My achievements are mostly volunteer things; I like to help people. Basically I have solved a lifetime of problems and have tried to raise my kids to be good citizens, to be problem-solvers, and to help other people. Unfortunately, my kids and I have all gotten hooked on giving a little too much to others and not concentrating on ourselves enough.

Generally I am happy with myself. But I wish other people would see that I have a humorous side! I guess it comes out only with my friends. Other people take me very seriously and evidently are intimidated, which I didn't realize. Strangers take me as a serious, confident person but they don't see the funny side of me. My friend Marsha says she sees me not so much as a person who is funny in and of myself but that I recognize and appreciate humor in other people. She says it takes a lot to make me laugh outright, but that I smile a lot. Maybe I have actually become more serious than I ever thought I was. Or maybe it's just that I worry about a lot of things. When we go on vacation, I have a good time; I enjoy Jerry and we have fun. Issues are important to me, though. I can't believe people don't watch the televised analyses of politics and news. I can't believe people don't want to be informed!

P A M, 46:
teacher, amateur athlete

My first memory of myself as a child was of my jet-black hair. I wore it parted in the middle, with bangs, and it looked very Oriental. I had large brown freckles, mainly on my nose, and people sometimes made fun of my big mouth. Even though I laughed, it hurt my feelings. I was about 6 years old.

I had two sisters, one younger, one older. They always made fun of my big lips! And I, in turn, made fun of my overweight older sister. She called me Liver Lips and I called her Tubby Tomkins! We were 10 and 14 by that time.

As I got older, I have memories of my very large "top," which was way out of proportion to the rest of my body. By the time I was 16 I was large-busted but small-boned and self-conscious. Unlike a lot of my friends, who wore sweaters over pointed bras full of tissue paper, I was hunched over like Quasimodo! My breasts probably weren't that large, but they didn't seem to match the rest of my body.

As far as my personality traits, I was always considered a clown and a jokester. I loved making people laugh; I still do! A couple of my girl-friends kept telling me, "You should be a comedienne like Martha Raye!" Well, to me, Martha Raye was one of the homeliest women alive, but then she too had a big mouth. They insisted that I was hilariously funny and kept egging me on, so I actually thought about it seriously for ten minutes. I felt I was too shy. I could never get up on a stage and perform.

I was not a real beauty. I could not get the really cute boys. But then again, I wasn't really interested in boys in high school; I was more inter-ested in sports, even though it wasn't a popular thing for girls in those days. In high school I played volleyball; in college I took fencing, horse-back riding, tennis and golf. As a young adult, I realized I was a good athlete. I was willing to try everything and I was good at whatever I tried. Soon, I was newly married, had a child, and was into motherhood. I put my own interests and self-development on the back burner.

I think I married my first husband because my father told me not to. That was the first time my father had said no to anything, and as a 21-year-old, I was going to assert myself. I think my first husband married me because my father was a famous musician with his name on the marquee above a famous local hotel. The young man, who was from the East, saw this and probably saw dollar signs, too. We married each other for different reasons, I guess. Nine years later, it wasn't working, but we had two sons.

Seven years later I remarried and, at age 39, I gave birth to my third son. Six months later I had a breast reduction. It was something I should have had done when I was 20 instead of at the ripe old age of 40. I started jogging regularly and even ran two marathons! The new breasts should have been with my body all along! Physically, it was a great move on my part. It wasn't so much for vanity, but for my own comfort.

Since the first surgery was so easy and I wasn't afraid of the knife, I had my eyelids done to eliminate their droopiness. It was outpatient surgery and I was out in an hour. Then after the upper eyelid surgery, I decided to have my lower eyelids done, too. This was all my doing; my husband had never said anything about my appearance.

Even back in high school, I had always been extremely self-conscious about the bags under my eyes. I got enough sleep, so they weren't bags from being tired; they were just hereditary. My father had them as well. I just had puffy circles all the time and looked as if I had been up all night crying. I remember wearing thick Max Factor pancake makeup, just literally painting it on to cover the bags under my eyes and the brown freckles on my nose.

My eyes are taken care of now, and I am content with the way I look, but I would consider having my face lifted in the fairly near future. I have my mother's skin, and I remember that by about the age of 50, her skin was terribly wrinkled.

I have also had my teeth fixed. I had porcelain veneers put on them about two years ago. My teeth were okay, but one was chipped and they were getting discolored. So my dentist talked me into this and it was great—expensive, but worth it.

The things I have done to myself are not the result of a lifelong desire to change myself. The opportunity simply came along and we could afford it, so why not? My husband never felt I needed to fix myself. He has always been very complimentary of my looks and figure. I wanted to make the changes. The rehab work cost quite a bit, and now my husband teases me that I am certainly not the girl he married! I don't know if it's a search for happiness or if I should even care what I look like. I feel young, why not look young?

My personality is my best trait. That may sound boastful, but I am very comfortable going into a party and talking to strangers. I love people. My intellect would be my second best trait. I have to rank my achievements third, although I am a teacher and I am very happy with that. I have no desire to be a principal or a Ph.D. I am happy changing the world just a little bit with what I do. I don't have to make money to be satisfied; my self-esteem is not dependent on that. I am happy with the person I am today. My self-esteem is good. I feel competent to take care of myself; I don't have to be dependent on anybody else.

There is a slight gap between my mirror image and my self-image. My mirror image is that of a 46-year-old woman with three children. Although I am pleased with the mirror image, my self-image is younger and cuter. Sexy! Pert!

I find approaching 50, a half century, very frightening. The older I get, the more active I get physically. I am running more, playing more tennis. I'm fighting this old-age thing to the bitter end. I'll be doing marathons when I'm 80 just to prove that I am capable. Old age does bother me, but it's also true that you are as old as you feel. Although there are days when I feel awfully old, having an 8-year-old son helps keep me going. Yesterday we played catch and went bike riding in the woods. I can't sit down for a minute. So, mentally, I am young and I wish my mirror image were a little more compatible with my self-image.

The aging process? Oh, Lord! I bought a book on how to age gracefully—what to expect in each decade as you age. I think the main things are to keep my mind stimulated and constantly have new goals. I can't stagnate and think about the past; I have to constantly move forward with enthusiasm and curiosity. But I will fight the aging process to the bitter end! I definitely want to stay physically fit. My mother had the same physique I do, and she did not take care of it. She was a heavy smoker, heavy drinker, and didn't exercise. She died in her early 70s. I am convinced she could have lived another twenty years, had she taken care of herself. That was a different generation. Being physically fit wasn't a priority for her.

PATRICIA, 49:

law school student

During my childhood and adolescence I developed a negative self-image and felt very much like an outsider. There were two reasons for this: my precociously mature appearance and my premature assumption of adult responsibilities. My large-for-my-age size and my mature-for-my-age attitude set me apart from other children and, later, from other teenagers. My mother had died when I was in kindergarten, my father travelled five days a week, and a series of housekeepers "babysat" for my younger brother and me in my father's absence. For these reasons, I had no adult guidance in dealing with my emotional reactions to my negative self-image, my outsider status, and my resulting feelings of loneliness and isolation.

Being an outsider meant many things to me. It meant that I looked different: I grew much faster than my classmates. By the fourth grade I outweighed—by about forty pounds—the "little" boy who was my first "crush." By the sixth grade I had reached my adult height of 5' 2" and weighed 130 pounds. While I looked like a small adult, my friends still looked like growing children.

Being an outsider also meant that adults treated me differently, and, often, insensitively. One of my clearest memories of such insensitive treatment is from the fourth grade. My homeroom teacher, Mrs. Lane, had caused me pain and embarrassment throughout the school year; however, she outdid herself the day that musical instruments were assigned. I attended grade school in Saint Louis, Missouri, at a time when the public schools provided musical instruments for students. By the fourth grade, I was tiring of the tomboy image I had acquired due to my size and had decided to choose a demure and feminine instrument, like the violin. However, when the music teacher reached our classroom, the cello was the last and only instrument available for assignment. A skinny little boy, named Michael, raised his hand and asked to play the cello. But no, Mrs. Lane stepped in, dashing poor Michael's hopes and thoroughly humiliating me when she said: "No, no no! We need someone who is big enough to carry the cello home to practice it. We'll let Patty play the cello!"

As an outsider, I no longer fit in at home. About a year after my mother's death, my father became involved with the young woman who would become my stepmother. Susan, who was in her early 20s when Dad brought her home to meet us, was 25 years younger than Dad and only 14 years older than I was. She was a thin, little size 4 person, and very different from the other neighborhood mothers, who were middle-aged women with middle-aged faces and middle-aged figures. Although my brother and I were proud of how youthful Susan was, her svelte figure was a double-edged sword for me. Again, it emphasized the fact that I was different because the female role model in my life did not look and act like the other moms. By the time I was 11, I weighed more than Susan, which caused me to feel awkward and ugly. I spent a great deal of time wishing I could be as skinny and as pretty as Susan. Unfortunately, that time could have been channeled into developing my talents and thereby contributing to a positive, rather than a negative, self-image.

Not having a mother also contributed to my feeling like an outsider. One of the ironies of my life has been that, as Susan and I have aged, Susan has been identified by most people as my natural mother. Adding to the irony was the fact that Susan and my father had a daughter, Tina, a blond Farah Fawcett-type who looked less like her mother than I did. Susan and I shared a similar brunette coloring, a similar conservative and tailored sense of style, and, eventually, a similar short, athletic physique.

Finally, being an outsider meant, unbeknownst to me, that my differences created resentment within the stepfamily environment. Susan's family was always extremely focused on appearances, in every sense of that word. Years of therapy and years of positive comments from friends have helped me realize that my stepfamily focused on my differences in order to detract from my natural beauty. Although the members of my step-family were attractive people, they were not "beautiful people." They did, however, thrive on competition. My negative self-image left me without the necessary confidence to compete in their arena of appearances. As a matter of fact, I neither understand the concept of competition nor the tactics people might potentially use to undermine those whom they saw as competition. I made it very easy for the members of my stepfamily to exclude me; they simply emphasized my differences and discounted my assets.

Susan recently gave me some pictures of myself from that time, and I realize now that I was an extremely beautiful young woman; however, I did not embody the ideal of beauty that was prescribed during my Sandra Dee-era adolescence. In those years girls had to be really skinny with long, straight blonde hair. Although I desperately wanted to look like everyone else among my peers with braces and glasses as well as straight blonde hair, I had extremely curly, dark brown, uncontrollable hair, which never looked like anyone else's hair. Because I just didn't fit the image, I grew up feeling very ugly. And it didn't help that we spent a lot of time with my new stepmother's family, obsessed as it was with appearances and weight. I don't think Susan realized how her family made me feel. I give her credit for instilling in me the idea that one could look good, dress well, and flatter one's figure at any weight. Even so, I was always trying to emulate the wrong role model; I wanted to be like the other kids or be accepted by Susan's family, and physically I didn't fit in anywhere. As an adult, I finally came to understand that my stepfamily hadn't rejected me personally; they were a very tightly-knit group who didn't have feelings for anyone outside their immediate circle, even my father!

My stepmother's mother, whom I called Grandma, always encouraged me to lose weight. Yet, when Susan finally showed me those old photos, I realized I was gorgeous! There was really no reason for me to lose weight.

I can see clearly from my current perspective that I simply have a large bone structure compared with my stepmother's tiny-boned physique. But in this particular family, as well as among other girls with whom I grew up, everybody bought into the idea of reed-thinness. And because, in those days, Dad always went along with Susan, he too thought it would be a good idea if I lost weight. Compounding the problem was the fact that, long before exercise was fashionable, Dad insisted that we exercise frequently, so I weighed more because I was all muscle. It was nuts! My weight was always such a big issue!

No one ever commented on my face or features. My mother's side of the family was lost to me by then, but I remember people saying, "You look a lot like your father." Obviously, the girl who was big enough to carry the cello didn't find anything feminine or dainty about herself. Being told that I looked like my father was just devastating to me. All I ever saw in myself was ugliness.

Because I had developed a woman's figure at an early age, I couldn't wear teen clothes. During sophomore year in high school, I made the cheerleading squad, and although I had already lost ten pounds, I had to go on a 600-calorie diet to get into the teen size 12 uniform pants which were the largest size available. It wasn't that I was heavy; I just didn't fit into teen clothes.

Even my prom dresses set me apart from everyone else. Susan never went for the typical frou-frou prom dresses. Everyone at the junior prom was in crinoline; I was the only girl in an elegant tailored cocktail dress. Of course, Susan was right: at 5'2" and 130 pounds, I didn't look good in frou-frou and crinoline. But being different was uncomfortable because it wasn't a good different. As a teenager, I wanted to be like everyone else.

I dated in high school, but it didn't alter my feelings about my looks. Generally, the boys saw me as a friend; I was never date-type popular. Also, it was the virgin era and Susan believed that because she was a virgin when she married, I too had to remain a virgin. The virginity issue was not necessarily a religious thing with her but more of a cultural issue. She felt it was the only thing—or one of the only things—that girls had to offer. I was not promiscuous, nor did I want to be. I was so naïve I didn't even realize that other kids were experimenting with sex, cigarettes, and alcohol.

Mitch, my first real boyfriend in high school, who was a year older and ran with a fast crowd, finally got fed up with my ingenuousness. It was too embarrassing to him to date someone who would never "park." Wanting to do right by the now-married Susan and Dad was such a driving force that I never did anything to get into trouble. Because I wouldn't go along with the program, dating Mitch didn't last very long. Especially a guy who drove a hearse—a ready-made motel!

I spent two difficult years at the University of Wisconsin in Madison trying to figure out what a degree would do for me. I sensed something was wrong at the time, but it has taken me many years to recognize how difficult school must have been for me because I have only recently been diagnosed with an attention deficit problem. I left school and took a job as a flight attendant with American Airlines in San Francisco. My dad didn't want me to quit school, but the family wasn't shocked at the decision because my Aunt Kate worked for Eastern Airlines.

I am glad I worked for American as a young woman because of the travel; I would never have lived that way in any other job. And given the job opportunities open to young women at that time it was not a bad choice. I would not have been happy teaching or nursing, so flying proved to be a very valuable experience. The downside was trying to maintain the required weight, which was completely unrealistic for my large bone structure. The airline wanted me at 105 pounds for 5'2". They were very strict in those days; any time my weight went over 110, they put me on weight check, which was constantly.

I also realize now that I have multiple food allergies. Back then I couldn't understand why one meal would make me gain three pounds. Unfortunately, I was dieting and eating incorrectly during the five years I flew, and I spent the whole time still feeling ugly.

Finally, when I could no longer keep my weight below 110 with diet alone and had gone back for another weight check after dieting and swimming madly, I was still three quarters of a pound over the limit. My supervisor threatened to take me off the line and insisted I would never fly for another airline again. I took her threat as gospel and also believed her when she said they would put me into a ground job. But six weeks later American went on a massive strike, laying people off, and putting a freeze on ground jobs.

When the American strike ended I was notified that I was eligible to start training for ground reservations. In order to be cleared for training, I had to go out to the airport for the required physical. The confused doctor gave me a flight physical instead of a ground physical. In addition, he made me and the forty pounds I had gained since my layoff parade around the room naked, while telling me it was a sin for a woman my age to look so grotesque. At that point I decided I could never work for the airline again. That decision put me in complete disgrace, as far as I was concerned, because I had already quit two other jobs thinking I was lined up for the American ground job. I went home, looked at the want ads, and got a job as a secretary in an ad agency.

It was at this point that I started running into trouble because of my looks! Despite my poor self-image and negative experience with the airline, I started to realize I was, in fact, fairly good-looking. During that time I held a series of office jobs that, for several reasons, did not last. First, I was quite independent and had never had to deal with authority. Up to this point I had been in control of everything I did; even as a child I had been in charge of the house and my brother. Second, as a secretary in an office where men were making what I viewed as ridiculous decisions, I went crazy; I ended up confronting them about their decisions. I assumed they wanted my input. It was havoc! There was no sexual harassment at the ad agency, but at every other job after that there arose the "new problem." And each succeeding job became impossible.

However, I did begin to take real pride in my newly realized creativity after I met my future husband, John. When I started living with him, I suddenly had more money to spend on clothes. I soon realized I loved clothing and what could be done with it, but I was also bored with the way everybody else put themselves together.

Once I started experimenting, my sense of style developed very rapidly. I didn't know the term "wearable art" at the time, but that is the style I created for myself even before I went back to school to work on my bachelor's degree in clothing and textiles. In the process of researching some of my course work, I discovered the whole field of wearable art clothing. I still wasn't convinced of my physical attributes, but I took great pride in putting clothes together because I felt so creative.

And for the first time in my life, my weight took a back seat, becoming less of an obsession. It truly became a non-issue unless it prevented me from putting together an outfit. I came to take pride in my appearance as an expression of my creativity. I so enjoyed putting clothes together with originality that I was surprised when other people failed to understand my style and often made fun of it. And yet I really didn't care what anyone else thought.

Basically I am comfortable with myself. The realization that I will be 50 in a year and a half has given me a wonderful feeling of empowerment. I feel my looks are better than ever now because, as I age, I am more comfortable with myself and my appearance. I reached a point several years ago when I was so comfortable with myself that everything else was icing on the cake. It was a tremendous period. But life has a way of handing me new challenges to shake me up. So I have to keep repeating the process to get back to the point I had reached before my breast cancer surgery last year. I had never accepted illness before because no one had ever allowed me to be sick. I have had to learn to accept the limitations of severe illness and what I can and cannot control.

Aging is very much on my mind because my father's life is being sustained in a way it shouldn't, and an elderly aunt is terrified of living on her own. Watching my husband face a forced retirement has made me see how much he is aging. I am only 48 and I feel a lot older than I should. I have had cancer so young; I just want this stage of my life to go away! I will have to face my own aging soon enough, and I feel I shouldn't have to deal with so serious an issue right now. Aging should be a mellowing process, but I don't want to deal with it. I certainly don't want it to influence my decisions in a way that makes me feel too old to do something new. It's starting to get to me and I don't think it's going to change; I think that's the way life goes. When I was younger and hadn't had a major illness I thought anything was possible, but once my life was threatened I realized everything isn't possible. I need to enjoy life while I've got it.

To defeat my alcoholism, I joined a lot of alcohol self-help groups which are very big on positive feedback. Recovering from alcoholism is a lesson in being totally honest with yourself. Many alcoholics never fully recover because they play games. But the groups I joined were so honest and positive that I can't imagine not having that in my life. It's a comment on the human spirit and on the strength of women. I shudder to think what my life would have been like without therapy and groups. Yet I am amazed that so many women don't share their struggles with each other. I give so much credit to those women who are not engaged in support groups for figuring out all those things on their own. But isn't it sad to reach 50 years of age before being able to affirm yourself and to have affirming people in your life?

Lately I have wondered how others perceive me. Law school has taught me to look at things from all sides. I get so excited about my own feelings and insights into myself that I often forget to think about how other people might feel about me. One of the women in our sobriety group once said to me, "Pat, one of the things that amazes me about you is that with all the shit going on around you, you just steer your own course and get it done. You just keep moving ahead through it all." I wondered during the cancer episode if I would ever be that strong again. My friend Terry, who is not open with her feelings and whose supportive stuff for others often comes out backhanded, commented that I need to realize that everyone is not as strong as I am. So I gather that others see me as very strong and stubborn yet compassionate and sympathetic. I attribute that to the fact that, although my upbringing with my stepmother encouraged me in a very passive role, I later sensed what was wrong with that behavior and worked to overcome it.

I use clothes as a powerful tool. I have no experience in dressing for business, but I always dress up to shop for designer sale items because I want store clerks to take me seriously as a collector. I don't want them to overlook a great piece in the back room because they think I am not a serious buyer.

I've not seen anyone put different styles together like I do. People in L.A. use clothes as a thrill-seeking addiction to get attention; New Yorkers tend to dress for status. When my friend Marge and I are in New York, a famous fashion photographer follows us around to various events and takes photographs of us. The photos are not always in the paper because we aren't wealthy, but he is always very interested in how we look. Marge and I are a pair of soulmates when it comes to creative personal style and we have a great deal of fun together!

I was finally able to make sense out of how different I felt during my life when, after flunking out of law school twice, my brilliant 72-year-old female oncologist diagnosed my attention deficit disorder. Attention deficit disorder has impacted every area of my life; however, the diagnosis was a true gift! It provided me with the answers I needed to move forward, proudly, with the rest of my life. Now, I truly understand all that I have to offer.

POSTSCRIPT: With the proper academic accommodations, I graduated from law school and passed the bar examination on my first try, in the top 10 percent!

PATTY, 44:

full-time wife and mother

I have a few recollections of myself as a child. When I was a little girl, I was so narrow in the hips that my mother always had to buy me boys' pants and shorts. I don't remember that particularly bothering me; it was a neutral experience. But at age 13 I was to be confirmed in a July ceremony, and I really wanted a particular sleeveless dress. Unfortunately my arms were so skinny I looked ridiculous in it, so I had to get a dress with sleeves. As a result, I never wear sleeveless things, even though I am no longer sensitive about my arms.

I also remember an incident in Wisconsin at our summer cottage. We were standing by the lake talking, when our neighbor came over. I was barefoot in a bathing suit, and he commented on how big my feet were for a kid. I'm a slight person, but I do have big feet and that has always bothered me. I still remember him saying, "God, she's got such big feet!" Being thin and having big feet—what a combo!

As a 14-year-old high school freshman, I went to London with my family for two weeks, when Carnaby Street was "in." I was hell-bent on a hip-hugger skirt. I could pass on the boots, but I had to have the hip-hugger skirt. We went to Carnaby Street to shop for one, but couldn't find one that would stay up! They all fell off me. That was an individual and personal experience, not related to anyone else. I don't have any memories of comparing myself with other people.

I grew up in an old established suburb of a large midwestern city, in one of the few Jewish families in our township. In general my parents were complimentary of my appearance, so I always felt good about my looks. During my teen years, I felt better than just okay about my looks. I was usually considered pretty cute, but I wasn't classic cute; I wasn't WASP homecoming queen, or even homecoming court. I wore braces on my teeth for a while, but a lot of the kids did, so that didn't really bother me. I dealt with my hair by ironing it; hair had to be straight in those days, and my hair isn't perfectly straight. It wasn't a traumatic thing, though. I don't even remember a very tough puberty. Maybe I was a terrible teen; I don't recall.

In high school I really didn't like my knees and I did compare them with the cheerleaders' knees. They all had great legs. I still don't have great legs; they are thin, but they are not beautifully shaped or toned, and they don't tan really well. But in general I felt very comfortable about my looks and relied on them maybe too much. I have attributed a lot of my social and professional success to the fact that I was reasonably attractive in terms of my physical being and personality. I always met people easily and had lots of men and women friends. I have always had good positive reinforcement about myself.

In high school I always had a lot of clothes, so people envied my wardrobe. When I was a young adult, women said they wished they could be as thin as I was. Men, too, were flattering to me. I am glad I kept the compliments in perspective because I wasn't a goddess. I was just fortunate to have avoided acne and bad chicken pox scars. My skin was always nice.

At one point in my life I was about 30 pounds heavier, but I was never heavy. Over the years I lost the weight and now I am stuck being thin. At 104 pounds, I am trying to put on some weight—10 pounds would do good stuff for me! During both of my pregnancies, people said that I looked really good, that it was a good time for me. My face is really thin now, along with my arms and legs and everything else.

I have had some negative comments on my voice as nasal and monotone. In college, I went on a European trip and some Europeans asked, "Is this what people from Chicago sound like?" I have always been aware that my voice is not a beautiful, soft, gentle, feminine voice. It is low and nasal and monotone, although it certainly never inhibited my talking or my behavior.

Later, when I quit teaching, my first job in the business world was in telemarketing. The job interview went fine, but the company vice president said, "I am sure you could do the job, and you're articulate. But

your voice! I just don't know that it would be good for telephone sales."
In that first interview he asked if I would be open to the idea of voice lessons.
And I said, "Yes, I don't really like my voice either." The vice president
was supposed to arrange for the voice lessons, but after I got the job, the
issue never came up again. But that was a heavy-duty comment.

I am increasingly aware of how lucky I have been because my complexion
and my hair never needed a lot of attention. I had good skin and thick,
robust hair that I didn't have to fuss with. I just depended on my natural
attributes. I am still not a primper—I am in and out of the locker room
at the tennis club in 10 minutes. I don't wear makeup, and I don't attend
to myself very much. But lately I feel I need to enhance myself more
because I am aging. I never really got into that stuff, so it's hard to suddenly try to put it into my daily routine. Friends insist that I always look
"together," that I look like someone who spends time on herself. Well,
that's good, because I take all of 10 minutes to get ready to go to an
important event.

Talking about the psychology of appearances, when I first started my
own telemarketing consulting business, I was so nervous that for the first
two weeks I got up in the morning and put on my navy blue business suit
to make phone calls from home to potential clients. I made it a point to
sit at my desk, or to stand to talk on the phone for these business calls.
Several weeks later I found myself making a business call lying on the sofa
with one leg hooked over the back, wearing shorts and a T-shirt! That's a
long way, baby!

I think that both my mirror image and my self-image have diminished in
the past few years. I gave up my career to marry and raise a family, even
though my career was a huge chunk of my self-image. I think most women
who give up their career and their sense of accomplishment and creativity
feel that way. I thrived on my accomplishments, and when I lost all those
positive strokes, I lost ground. My young daughter doesn't say, "Great meal,

Mom." The wife-mother job is just not acknowledged. Trying to keep up with a very busy, active, successful husband and two very small, active children is very tiring. It has its positive moments, but it's not all positive.

For most of my life, others' perceptions of me were very much in line with my own. I always felt good about myself, that I was accomplished and capable. I have always been successful in putting my message across, getting a job, or getting clients for my consulting business. But there is definitely a gap between my perceptions and others' perceptions of me now.

Last week I had dinner with an old friend and when I told her about my diminished sense of self-image, she was in shock! She couldn't believe that I felt this way about myself. Obviously, other people don't see me as I see myself right now.

Whether it's paid work or avocation or involvement, I need to get back into the swing of accomplishments. I can't just car pool and be at my family's beck and call. I wish it were satisfying for me. I just don't feel good enough about myself doing that stuff exclusively. I see myself doing something in the business world again—I had hoped by next fall, but it won't be that soon. My youngest, my son, will still be a baby. And I don't want to miss these early years with the children. Given that choice, I will probably feel bad about myself for a while, in order to be with the children. I feel too torn when I am away. It's hard to concentrate on telemarketing issues, compared with being with my kids. Maybe if I were a doctor or lawyer it would be different.

The aging process has taken a toll on my physical being and it bothers me. I don't feel as comfortable with myself now. I look dragged out and the grey hair doesn't help. I am tired and the fatigue is a big part of it. When people call you "ma'am" and not "miss," that's a sure sign you are aging!

Recently my husband and I went to an art gallery event. As we were leaving, a woman rushed over to us and said the owner wanted to know who those people in their 40s were! It was obviously a real young crowd that night. So we are getting older and it's bothering me more than I ever thought it would, because my feelings about my looks were always very strong and positive.

I don't have a plan for dealing with the aging process, and I think everybody should have a plan. As an older parent of very young children, I think it's important to have a personal approach to aging. My son is only 19 months old. When he wants to romp around, play in the grass, throw a ball, learn to ride a bicycle without training wheels, who is going to run after him? I will have to do that in a wheelchair! I will have to have an exercise regimen just to stay even with the aging process. I play tennis. I try to exercise a couple times a week—the Nordic Track or running, if it's nice out.

To me, the key is to maintain my mental health in the chaos of domestic engineering—to retain a sense of self-respect and accomplishment. I think women who have done well in their careers are less likely to succumb to these feelings of diminished self-image. To me that's most important—nurturing that feeling of accomplishment.

R E N E E, 35:
physical therapist

I grew up in South Africa. I don't recall much of my childhood; there are a lot of gaps. However, I recently went into therapy, and interesting stuff is coming up. I've asked my mother and brother to enlighten me on some things, but I still have big patches of missing memories.

My mother said she always tried to dress me in the morning, and I refused her assistance. There was no way I was going to wear Mother's choice. Although I preferred pants and never liked skirts or dresses, there was a pinafore dress that she always wanted me to wear. I remember it clearly and I hated the damn thing. But I wore it sometimes just to avoid a confrontation.

Growing up, I never went shopping with my mother. She had no clue as to what I liked to wear. She tried to dress me in what she liked to see me in. She finally gave up buying dresses for me, but even when she tried she couldn't pick out a sweatsuit for me! I remember one birthday she bought me a warm-up suit in rust, beige, and brown—my worst colors! I was 23, and I said, "Mom, you've lived with me for 23 years, surely you'd know I am not going to wear a brushed velvet, rust-and-brown sweatsuit."

As a kid I was a tomboy and into sports. I remember climbing a lot of trees and skateboarding with my brother, my only sibling. I don't remember getting any feedback from either of my parents about sports. It was cool with everybody. I was beyond the pinafore dress by then, just wearing jeans, T-shirts, shorts, and bathing suits.

My growing sense of self-image? Apparently when my brother was born three years after me, my father rejected me. It probably wasn't a conscious thing, but here finally was the son that he had always wanted. And he showered all his affections on my brother. I can remember my father coming home from work, holding his arms out to my brother. My mother tells me she would say, "Dear, you have a daughter as well." My brother remembers that also. Apparently this went on for some time. I may have been aware of it then, and blocked it out. My brother remembers many times when my father would give him things, or say nice things to him, and he would think, "Oh, I hope Renee doesn't get upset!" I have no recollection of this, however.

I have spoken about this to my psychotherapist because one of my physical therapy patients once asked me if I had been a tomboy when I was younger. And I said, "Yes, I was and I think I always have been." And then we got into this thing about my being rejected by my father, and how I may have dressed like my brother to be a boy that my father wanted. I never felt unloved by my parents; they loved us both and told us so. But those things definitely played a role in my self-image.

I can't remember how I saw myself in my teen years. I had a lot of friends and was confident and outgoing. I always needed positive feedback from other people, however—a trait I have had from a very early age. I still have my nursery school reports, which say I needed positive reinforcement from my teachers all the time. I'm still like that today. I either ask for feedback directly, or I go about getting it in subtle ways.

I went to an all-girl's high school and had a lot of close friends from whom I got mostly positive feedback. Yet I remember some very insecure times with my friends, also. For years, I was inseparable from Dana, a close friend; but if she made plans with someone else, I took it really personally. And when I was at university, the same thing would happen with my best friend Karol.

My high school friend Dana and her mother had a wonderful relationship. I remember wanting that same closeness with my mother. I'd even say to myself "Okay, now I am going to go home and try!" But I knew that it really wasn't there, and it wasn't going to be there. I think I spent more time at Dana's house than mine. I'd ride my bike there after school, and then try to get my mother to allow me to sleep over on a week night! She always said no.

And every Saturday morning Dana and I took the bus downtown and went shopping. I was jealous of her wardrobe; she had great clothes, and lots of them. She always dressed in nice pants, whereas I wore jeans everyday.

Young adulthood was a very confusing time for me. I started my university studies and left, and then didn't know what I wanted to do. I went to New York, and then came home. I worked for a newspaper. I changed a lot of things about myself. I had never had a wonderful relationship with my mother, and the differences between us became more apparent at this stage because I was living at home. My mother felt I was just a boarder in the house; I was always going somewhere and doing something. She hated the fact that I enjoyed myself and had few responsibilities. I kept getting the message from my mother that I had to be more responsible. Maybe it was all her insecurity projected on me.

During the past three years away from home, I've done about a 180-degree turnaround. I am so much more aware of who I am. I still have a lot of the same issues, but they are so much easier to deal with now. And I understand where I am coming from. I am just so much more open. It saddens me to think about how I was then—so uncommunicative with everybody, even my closest friends. I was more communicative with them than I was with my mother, but nothing compared with now. So those were the biggest changes: getting away from home, distancing myself from my family, getting into therapy, and finding a sense of direction and a career path. And the most important factor was confronting my sexuality, which obviously governs who I am now. It's such an important part of who I am and how my life has changed in the past three years.

I have no confusion with who I am now. I am pretty clear about what I want in my life as far as my relationships are concerned, and I am clear about my sexuality. But then I never went through a period of intense confusion: Am I a lesbian? Am I not a lesbian? It just happened, and the transition was pretty easy. And it's made it so much easier to get on with the other stuff. The reason I went into therapy was not because I was confused about my sexuality; in fact I deal with it very little in therapy because it's not an issue to me at all. The reason I went into therapy was to find out who I am, and what it's all about. I only just realized how important it was to get away from home and away from my family. I needed to be away to find out who I am and where I am going.

I dated a lot in high school and college, but although I went out with great guys, I got bored six weeks down the line. I just never formed any close personal attachments to any of them, to my father, or to any other men. So I'd break up with these great guys and regret it afterwards, but I know now there was never anything there. With my women friends there is definitely an emotional attachment!

Dealing with my sexuality while living in the small Jewish community within my hometown was problematic because you were expected to get married and have kids. In getting out, I realize that there is no way I could go back and live like that. I think if I had stayed in my hometown, I would never have gotten to this stage. I don't think I would have even gone into therapy, much less make any of the other changes I've made.

My relationship with my mother is so much better now, just because I am so much more accepting of myself and my sexuality. It has made a really big difference. I wish now that my mother and I could spend time together. There would be so much more tolerance.

I think I always had a positive perception of my appearance. Although I always got negative feedback from my mother about the way I dressed, I felt good about what I was wearing and how I looked. It was comfortable to me. I don't remember ever being unhappy about my appearance.

We had to wear uniforms in grammar school and high school. That was the best thing in the world: I didn't have to wake up every morning and worry about what to put on. Even through physical therapy school we wore uniforms, which happened to be flattering to my coloring, so dressing was always easy.

I never wore makeup; I was too lazy and didn't know how to go about it anyway. My mother and most of my friends wore makeup, but it didn't interest me. I never got negative feedback from my parents about my physical appearance. My boyfriends told me that I had a good figure or that I was pretty, and my friends said the same things. I never had destructive, competitive relationships with my friends; there were always compliments. I was lucky in that way.

My job as a physical therapist doesn't require dressing up; it requires ease of movement and comfort. I know a lot of people who are insecure but dress to project a confident image. They really dress up or wear expensive stuff. I am not interested in dressy clothes, yet I am very stylish and current. Yeah, I go to the Gap every week! I know what's out there. I do a lot of shopping! And I have an incredible amount of clothes and spend a lot of money on my wardrobe even if it's very casual.

What words best describe my most positive mental image of myself? I always knew that I had a decent body, tall and thin, with long legs. And I consider myself attractive—not a world-class beauty, but I know I am pleasing to look at. I give off a confidence and positive energy that enhances the physical. I would never look at myself in the mirror and think bad things!

Generally the feedback I get matches my own perceptions of myself. A few times at university, when I was introduced to new people, I later got some feedback that they found me very aloof and unfriendly. And that really disturbed me. I think sometimes I'm seen as having an attitude because, if I don't know somebody or if I'm in a new crowd, I may just sit back and survey the scene. And because I am quite confident and have a lot to say for myself, people can be put off, I suppose. But generally the feedback I've gotten is that I am friendly, outgoing, interested in other people, and a good listener. As a freelance physical therapist, I always look forward to meeting new colleagues and patients.

I am happy with the person I am today, happier than I have ever been, and more aware of myself. In the future, I would like to get rid of what insecurities I have and just keep changing as life goes on. I must say that I looked forward to turning 30, because women are in their prime—and even more so after 40! I look forward to each day, although it upsets me that the years are going so quickly.

I don't have any clues as to dealing with the aging process, let alone next month or next year. I deal with the here and now, not the future. A lot of people my age have more direction than I do. I am not direction-less, but my mother would probably still call me irresponsible. I still go out and have fun and spend my money. And I'm not ambitious enough to open up my own practice and make $250,000 a year. I am very happy working eight hours a day, going to movies every night, and being able to travel or pick up and move to a new location.

I have a pair of wild shoes that I got here in the States. They look like dressy mountaineering boots, and I love them. But when I took them home with me and put them on for my mother, she said, "Ugh! Those are boy's shoes!" It wasn't how she wanted to see me—not what she expected. I brought them back to the States and now when I wear them, all my friends love them!

ROBERTA, 52:
psychiatric nurse

As a tomboy child I had to wear corduroys and I didn't like that. I wanted to dress prettily like a girl, but I also wanted to climb trees. My sister Marie, three years older and the "beautiful" one, got to wear dresses.

One time, my mother had made me a beautiful dress out of that white sheer stuff with little purple violets all over it. I thought, "I'm going to be very careful with this dress and I'm not going to tear it or get it dirty, or anything!" Then I went and sat on the neighbors' swing and the dress caught on a splinter and tore. I wanted to die!

I was the second daughter, named after my father. Because I knew Dad had always wanted a son, I kept trying to be that little boy. Keeping up with the neighborhood kids made me even more boyish, because the other kids were tough. Everybody just ran loose in our neighborhood. I was always the smallest and youngest, and since I was also short and chubby, I was always running to keep up. Falling into things. Falling out of things. Even if I tried not to, I still got hurt. One of the teenage neighbor kids often used my cousin Jimmy and me for guinea pigs, making us box each other or using us for target practice with his BB gun!

Some of the neighborhood boys once dropped a noose around my neck and briefly hanged me from their garage roof. Another time, the really nasty boy next door hit me right between the eyes with a hammer, breaking my nose and blackening both my eyes. One summer day somebody in the group shoved me from a garage roof and gave me a compression fracture. Another day, my cousin Jimmy threw a rock which hit a telephone guywire, ricocheted back, and chipped my new front tooth just coming in. That summer I was black and blue from head to toe—bloody, bruised, bandaged—and running around trying to keep up with the big guys!

I could get hurt all by myself, too. Jumping from the neighbors' garden bench to their birdbath, I missed and fell into a pine tree. Ran a branch into my eye! The stick punctured my eyelid, causing a horrible mess. I got horrendously damaged all the time. So, by age 6, I saw myself as a messy, grubby little kid, who was inadequate to the task of surviving in our neighborhood.

Healthwise, I never simply got sick: I always just about died. I didn't get a cold: I got pneumonia. I didn't get scarlet fever once: I got it twice! One summer, I had a blood disorder which caused every mosquito bite to hemorrhage. The doctor thought I had leukemia because of all the bruises from the mosquito bites. My mother would just say, "Oh my God!", and go on to the next crisis; although, to her credit, she tried hard to civilize me, the little barbarian.

I couldn't do anything with my hair. In grade school, my mother put my hair in French braids. The day I hurt my eye, one of the braids had come undone. My whole head was bandaged for six weeks with the one braid unbraided. My mother was probably more upset about that braid than the possibility of my losing movement in my eye. Her major concern was: what would people think about my unbraided hair?

My dad went into the service when I was 4 and was away all the time. I knew Dad liked my sister best because he called her "Angel" and he called me "Picklepuss." I didn't like that. However, my Uncle Henry, who lived down the street, always liked me better than my sister Marie. He thought I was wonderful; he still gets a kick out of my feistiness.

Until sixth grade, I was short and chubby and didn't yet see myself as a girl. However, my sister had already blossomed into full womanhood and was truly striking. Everyone thought she was gorgeous. Because Marie was so striking, people would stop us on the street and say, "Oh, what a beautiful girl." And then they would turn to me and say, "You look just like your mother." And I would think, "Oh, shit," because my mother was not pretty. When I was about 16, the guy who worked at the bus station said, "Your sister is beautiful. What happened to you?" I remember laughing and saying, "Somebody goofed," even though I felt just awful.

Because my sister was beautiful but quiet and underachieving, I cultivated my personality, intellect, and accomplishments. By the teenage years, I had a much better sense of myself as an excellent student who was very intellectually competitive. However, I had no sense of my femininity. By then I was quite tall; in one year I had grown six inches—all in my legs. As a result, I became very self-conscious about those long legs. I didn't see myself as physically attractive. When one of the guys started calling me "Legs," I immediately took it negatively. A lot of those comments were really compliments, or clues that I was okay, but I just didn't pick up on them.

When the captain of the football team asked me to a formal dance, my sister's current boyfriend asked me how I was going to hold up my yellow strapless formal. I said, "You don't need to worry about that. I'm not going with you!" I had adopted this kind of cold, cynical, sarcastic way of dealing with males because they scared the living daylights out of me.

In high school, I grew to 5' 8". I wanted to be shorter because most of the girls were shorter. My best friend Joanne was little, a cheerleader, and tanned easily. I fantasized about getting a disease that would shrink my bones, turn my hair blonde and my eyes green, and cause me to tan.

During my teen years I wanted to be sexy. At 13, I started working and buying my own clothes but it was very difficult for me to get anything to fit because of my height. And I still saw myself as a dud. By the time I got into high school, most of my girlfriends were dating and I was not. I went out once in a while but I just didn't feel very sexy.

My parents were divorced when I was 13, and I continued to overachieve, to be the family hero. My sister was acting out and had horrendous fights with my mom. And my mother would say to her, "You're acting like a female!" So I thought, "You can't be sexy, a girl, or female. And you're not doing very well as a boy; you keep getting hurt. You'd better just stick with the intellectual stuff because that's all you're good at."

Then I found out about model samples at a trunk show at my favorite dress shop. The woman in charge asked me to try things on and walk around the store in them. She outfitted me in some very sharp clothes, with high heels and all the accessories. She put me together and I really enjoyed it. Suddenly people paid attention to me. That was neat. Those samples really fit me. That was the first glimmer that maybe I was not as ugly as I thought, compared with my gorgeous older sister.

During teenage years and high school, my sister and I were both in Rainbow Girls, the teenage girls' division of the Masonic Eastern Star. Formal meetings required formal gowns—and thanks to those model samples, we had some great dresses. Both Marie and I probably looked stunning in those evening gowns, but I was competing with an older sister who ultimately became a model. (Mom kept telling her, "You'd better hang on to your looks, because you haven't got a brain in your head!") Now I just wish I had appreciated the body and the looks that I had back then!

My dream was to go to college and become an English teacher, but I couldn't afford it. With a Kiwanis scholarship I could afford nurses training. For three straight years, summers included, the cost was only $1,000 with room and board.

In nursing school, I did better socially, although my height was a drawback at the local college mixers. One 5' 6" guy said to me, "My God, you're tall," and then he turned around and walked away. That meat market situation at mixers was very offensive. Part of me felt inadequate, but part of me said that guys should not treat women this way.

But in my nursing studies, I felt very competent. Nurses training was very real and I just settled in and got comfortable. During our brief summer vacation, when I saw my old friends who had gone to college, I could no longer relate to them. I was dealing with life and death; they were dealing with fraternities and sororities. I take life more seriously, always have. I wish I weren't like that but I am.

My freshman year in nursing school there was a big beach party and I went because I liked to swim. What did I know? I couldn't believe the other gals wore padded strapless bras and panty girdles under their bathing suits. I was a genuine swimmer; I didn't do any of that. I thought it was the strangest thing!

Living with all those women at school exposed me to lots of different levels of feminine development. There were some people who were even more innocent and naïve than I was. And then there were girls living with guys and doing things so they wouldn't get pregnant. That was another type of education.

In those days I was self-conscious about my big hips and wore a girdle even under Bermuda shorts. There we all were flattening out the bottom and wearing ice-cream-cone bras on the top to compensate. By the time I was midway through nurses training I had dated a lot of guys. I was actually feeling feminine and learning about the sexual part of my nature. One guy I dated made every erotic zone vibrate, but my Catholic upbringing always reminded me, "You could go to hell for that."

Those were pretty good years. And I finally met Jim, settled down, and got married. That was thirty years ago and I have gone through a lot of changes in self-image from career-oriented, to wife, to the jock thing. Jim and I skied and raced small sailboats. Jim always said if I weren't so concerned about being a lady, I'd be a good tennis player! Most of that jock stuff I did for him; I don't think I'm very well-coordinated. Mother always said I was a klutz and I believed her!

Being part of a young married couple was a pretty neat new thing. We had a lot of fun. I worked a couple of more years, we had our first baby, and then we bought a house. Talk about appearances! Jim couldn't stand the sight of me pregnant. He hated fat women and still does.

I started taking oil painting classes when I was pregnant the first time. My sister Marie took classes too, and was always better than I was at all the things I thought were important. (I could out-think her, but that wasn't important in my mind.) I didn't even think I could draw, but when I started art classes I discovered some talent. The art teacher was very helpful, bringing books for me and encouraging my budding skills. I began to do paintings every bit as good as my sister's.

That was probably my most authentic time: reading, painting, planting flowers, raising kids, and keeping a home. Everything seemed well-balanced. One day, when our minister came by to ask if I would help the local kids with a drug program, I went back into nursing again. I was ready to crusade and ended up investing a lot of energy in that program. I put everything I had into living. I was 31, and 30 had been a rough birthday for me. I had thought, "What am I gonna do now?" That drug center was what I was going do!

Initially, I didn't know anything about street drugs. Those local kids taught me about them. And we had just gotten the program's funding proposal passed when Jim and I were transferred out of town with his company. I never saw the building go up for my program! But I was awfully proud of what we did. There was a lot of ego stuff for me in that work. Working with people toward a common goal was a thrill.

Over the past ten years, as my physical appearance has deteriorated, I have become more concerned about my looks. I was always thin, but since my hysterectomy a couple years ago, I have gained weight that I cannot take off. No matter what I do, I can't lose it. That's very difficult for me partly because my mother was fat and I found it repulsive. And I can't figure out what to do about it. Should I keep trying to fight this weight, or should I go with the size I am and dress for it? I have not wanted to buy all new clothes in size 12 or 14, so I've just bought a couple of outfits. I have a lot of trouble now with the weight issue and with losing my physical strength due to back problems. In my teen years I coped by using my intellect and sarcasm, but that's going too! Aging is a matter of constantly adjusting to new stuff.

I would rather not have wrinkles, but that's all the laughter and all the tears and all the sunshine of 50 years of living and I wouldn't have missed any of it. It's okay, being wrinkled. But being fat is not! I don't like being overweight, having these little rolls and cellulite that's reaching critical mass. In my youth I was flat-chested and always wanted a bust. Well, now I have a bust but I also have a tummy! I just have to balance the stuff out in my mind.

Although I don't like to change my looks very much, experimenting with various appearance changes started with braces on my teeth. I had twelve congenitally missing teeth; my existing teeth were shifting very badly; there were bone and periodontic problems. I didn't really do the braces for cosmetic reasons but I do like the way it looks much better.

I am struggling with midlife issues—empty nest and a surgical menopause. But I have finally developed a sense of humor and a little lighter attitude. When we came back from our summer place last fall, my hair had turned a very brassy color. In an effort to tone it down with do-it-yourself hair color, I turned it plum-colored! There was a time when I would have called in sick rather than go to work with plum-colored hair. Well, I went to work and just kept saying, "It'll wash out. It's okay!" I am really comfortable enough with myself at this stage of the game.

Certainly, I don't think I look as good as I did ten years ago. I don't like the extra weight and I don't like having physical limitations. When my back gets bad and keeps me from walking or moving around, I get really depressed. The macho part of me would still like to go out and windsurf with Jim. But I am getting more comfortable without those things in my life.

So, these feelings about my looks have been a roller-coaster ride. But for me it's the balance of life that is important. One of the best things I ever did was take a trip to Ireland on my own a few years ago. I got a real sense of who I was without Jim, without the job, just going, being a part of a group, and having a marvelous time meeting a lot of neat people.

My job doesn't have the power it once had. And yet a lot of that has become more comfortable, too, because I no longer have to fight my overactive sense of responsibility. I often talk about the aging process with Tom, my friend and buddy at work. I recently told him that I now look better with clothes than without. He in turn commented on the magic of "corrective clothing" and then said, "We're suffering from incipient longevity!" I really need somebody around with that attitude.

R O S E, 48:
nurse

My first memory of my appearance as a child is in relation to Patty, the girl who lived across the street. I was about 5; she was my first friend and playmate. She was an only child, blonde and pretty, with cute clothes, and her own room. I can remember being over there with her and her parents, aware that I had long straight black braids and a fat little face and, of course, no fancy clothes. We had good times together, but I think of myself in contrast to Patty in those earliest memories, which are more distinct than any memories of being at home with my brothers and sisters.

I guess I always felt plain, not pretty or feminine, as I grew up. But it wasn't really a negative experience; I never felt badly. It was just an observation. I always felt very secure at home with my mother, so it didn't matter. I didn't seem to care what I looked like or stop to think about it, and I'm still that way.

I always got good grades both in elementary and high school, but I still never considered myself an exceptional student. I was not nominated for National Honor Society. I wasn't active enough or outgoing enough, and I think I was a little behind socially. I couldn't recite or give a speech, but I could get the grades on paper; I was really good at that.

Growing up, I always felt secure at home and with my friends. I had such nice friends in grade school and high school, who paved the way for my whole life. Because I was such a follower, I have often wondered what would have happened to me if they hadn't been such good kids, although in a few situations I felt uncomfortable with people doing things that weren't right. So I guess I wouldn't have strayed too far. But my friends always made me feel good.

In elementary school I was considered in the popular crowd, but the school was so small, there wasn't much else! The summer before seventh grade, all the girls voted me in as captain of the cheerleaders. I was really thrilled but also really nervous. It meant that for the coming school year, I was supposed to take charge, be innovative, take the initiative, and I couldn't do that. That experience made me realize I was different. Sure, I was a nice person, but I couldn't take charge; I didn't have what it takes to lead. The girls were aware of that, too, so they just kind of took over for me.

My brothers and sisters and I were all pretty close together in age, and we always had lots of friends playing at our house. And I always had boyfriends. In eighth grade, we switched boyfriends a lot, which was fun! In high school I didn't have a boyfriend for a couple of years, until junior year when I started dating Don. He was really nice and we dated through the rest of high school and a couple of years into my stint at nursing school. I broke that relationship off because something wasn't clicking.

And then a year or so after that I met Bill. During that transition time, I didn't feel I needed a boyfriend, but when I met Bill there was just something about him that made me feel good about myself. I didn't have to prove anything. Regardless of any other problems in the marriage, there has always been that feeling in our relationship. I guess I was very lucky because that really helped me feel good about myself and my decision-making abilities.

In high school, then, I felt secure but never as good as anybody else. I sat in study hall and watched the girls who were so pretty, so smart, so talented, and who could do all the things I felt I couldn't. And yet I didn't feel badly about myself, I just admired everyone else. I thought everyone else knew everything and could do everything better than I could.

I always admired my friend Maureen so much. She was completely without any airs and from a humble background, no big house or anything. But she was the neatest person. She was at ease with everybody; she knew everybody's name and remembered everybody. And I always wondered how she was that self-assured at such a young age. She taught dancing after school, got good grades, and was active in all the school musicals. She had so many roles and she was so good at them all. She just amazed me and I will always remember her!

When I got to nursing school, I started feeling good—well, better—about myself in terms of my own accomplishments. At first, I was very nervous, studied every minute, and was very conscientious about school. Once I was out of school and working, it still seemed as if it took me much longer than anyone else to get comfortable in my new role. But once I sensed my competency, it was marvelous to feel assured about what I was doing. Now, I can walk into a new patient's hospital room with his or her family present, and just take over and make them all feel at ease. But in a social situation or party, I'm just no good. I still cannot make easy social conversation! But I think that's the way it will always be, and I have accepted it. I am not the type to be captain of the cheerleaders or a social butterfly. That's how I am. At this point I am satisfied being a nice person with a few close friends and being good at what I do.

At my age, I feel I should do more in social circles like committee work or teaching catechism classes. But either I can't comfortably do those things or I just don't want to put in the effort. For a while I was on the board at the community center and I did a fairly good job there, but I have dropped out. When I was young and newly married and asked to do these things, I did them, and sometimes I felt it was too much. I may have been partially burned out on these activities.

In terms of my physical appearance, I don't look as good as I used to. I am wrinkled and a little gray; I don't take care of my face or my skin very well. I could do something about that easily enough, but I never have. It's not that important to me; neither is dressing well. So I don't think I look as good, but I definitely feel better about myself than I ever did, and that's more important.

I don't have a natural smile; all my life, my crooked teeth have discouraged me from smiling. That is why, in terms of my mirror image, I see someone with a very serious face. Without a natural smile, I think I look much more serious in the mirror than I really am, and I look older in the mirror than I really feel. I guess we all feel that at this age. When my dad turned 70 he said, "I can't believe it; I feel just like I did when I was in my 30s!" So I realize that age doesn't really change you inside—although sometimes I think I should act a bit more as if I am pushing 50. I could be just a bit more sophisticated!

As far as how others perceive me, nobody ever tells me they don't like me—although I have gotten a few greeting cards that say, "A friend is someone who knows all about you and likes you anyway!" I have gotten several of those and I wonder if they are trying to tell me something!

Some time after Bill and I were married and our daughter was small, Bill's 8-year-old son Benjamin came to live with us. That was when I became the evil stepmother in Benjamin's eyes. Bill and I were both constantly on Benjamin's case for his behavior, and naturally the boy's perception of me was very negative. This is the only time I am aware that I was cast in a bad light, and of course our relationship has changed over the years.

So, I don't really know how my peers perceive me. When I use my family as a sounding board, they always tell me that I put myself down too much. I don't know why it took me so long to develop a stronger self-image. I guess it's the fact that I'm so uncomfortable with social events, but I have come to terms with that as much as I can at this point in my life.

S A N D I, 25:
professional dancer

I really have no first memory of my appearance but, because I had no siblings, my parents are very strong in my recollections. They constantly gave me very positive reinforcement about everything—sometimes too much and to the point where it drove me crazy. But now I appreciate it.

I was a gymnast at a very young age, and was fortunate to have natural ability that got me a lot farther than most people. In high school I was one of the top gymnasts and got a lot of praise. All that stroking gave me a very good self-image, until I was shocked out of it by the real world of gymnastics. When I left home to further my gymnastic studies, I was one of the worst kids at the gym! However, my sensitivities had nothing to do with physical appearance or aesthetics, but with what my body could do in gymnastics. Although I had a lot of natural ability, I was one of the weakest gymnasts because my upper body strength was never what it should have been. That's probably why I am a dancer today and not a gymnast.

In my family, there was much emphasis on me as a person—no emphasis on my looks at all. I was given credit for putting together an outfit, or looking nice, but my parents would have been positive no matter what I put on. They acknowledged my appearance but they didn't dwell on it. They let me try anything, and if I failed, they let me decide to continue or not. I didn't have any siblings until I was out of the house, so I got lots of attention. They were always positive, always very supportive.

In my teenage years, however, I hated myself. That's when I became aware of my appearance. I felt my friends were much prettier. They always had the boyfriends. But then again, I was always at the swimming pool, the gym, or dance class, so I didn't have time. That might have had something to do with it, but at the time I didn't think so. I would spend hours trying to fix my hair and nothing ever worked. I would beg for a perm and after my mom spent the money for it, I would hate it and spend all my time brushing and washing and conditioning to restraighten my hair. There were some traumatic years in our house.

It has only been in the past five years that I have started to come out of my shell. Most of my formative years were spent with gymnasts or dancers while our teachers ripped us all to shreds. We were without confidence, not only in our ability, but also in our intelligence. They would say, "You're not smart enough to do this!" We all experienced tremendous negativity from the teacher, choreographer, or director, depending on the stage of our career. There has to be a better way to teach the arts. You don't achieve beauty in motion with such negativity; it's too destructive.

Maybe what really saved me was that I came to the experience with so much positive stuff from my parents. When I was very young and before I went away to study, they gave me a lot of affirmation and emotional support. They provided me with a much stronger sense of self than some of my other friends received. When many of my peers got into a destructive situation with no ability to resist, they were destroyed.

For me, much of my self-image during this time came from the pursuit of thinness. When I think about the first person who told me to lose weight, I could just kill him! He was a gym coach in California, where I was training. He was a superior being in my mind and, away from home at age 13, I trusted what he said. Of course he didn't tell me how to do it! He just said, "Lose weight." The reality was that I didn't need to lose weight, but his comment made me look in the mirror and reject what I saw. That's where it all started; since then 98 percent of my image has been my weight. Plus I was just about at the age when girls start to gain weight as a natural part of the maturing process, and because of the extreme dieting my metabolism got messed up. It wasn't until I was 22 that my stalled metabolism finally started to normalize.

The emphasis on thinness was widespread at the performing arts high school I attended, but there was no counseling or nutrition program to deal with it. One girl became so bulimic that she couldn't remember what happened two days ago, or even carry on a conversation. The last time I talked to her was five years ago; she was mentally gone. Other friends are currently very overweight because of those thinness issues in high school. Now I see how horrendous the situation was. Fortunately, I fixed myself. I realized one day, lying in bed so weak that I couldn't dance, that I was defeating the whole purpose of my life. So I decided to get straightened out. But if I'd had the help of a nutritionist that first time around I could have done it in a more civilized, educated, and healthy manner. I went from one extreme to another: crash diets, weight gains; smoking, not smoking; more weight gains, more futile diets. Not until I was finally given a recommendation to see a nutritionist did I get my weight under control in a healthy manner. As it turned out I needed only one visit with the nutritionist to find the correct information to change my way of life and my eating habits.

Fortunately, my body responded to the nutrition program and the new way of life. And my self-image has improved because I feel more normal. At one point I couldn't even remember what that felt like anymore. Of course, feeling out of control is one of the worst things for your self-esteem.

That's why, when I gain even a few pounds, I see myself as disproportionately big. I don't react like I used to, but I say, "Wait, I really have to get on top of this!" Like any addiction or disorder, it's always with you. Even if you have conquered active anorexia or bulimia and gotten back to a fairly normal weight, it is always in the back of your mind.

In high school, I had jaw surgery for improved alignment and comfort, along with some cosmetic adjustments to reduce the extra gum above my top teeth. I had been somewhat self-conscious about it, but I didn't know how much until I saw the great improvement after the surgery. That was a major appearance change but I didn't think about the aesthetic effect until it was over.

After the jaw surgery, and after I began working as a dancer, I started accepting my appearance as working for me. I had had long stringy ballerina hair until I joined a jazz dance company where everyone had short hair. I have since cut mine short; it's much more flattering to me.

The way others perceive me has always had to do with personality and ability. They have said: "She's so dependable, she's so reliable." That comment is certainly a compliment, but left-handed. I would like to be told that I look nice, too.

At this point, I am not dissatisfied with myself. I am "safe" in terms of my look. Everything still comes back to dancing: if I look okay for what I am doing, and I look good doing it, then I am okay with it. If I look in the mirror and it's okay, then I am okay. If I am repulsed by it, then I get a haircut or try something new with makeup.

My boyfriend of five years, with whom I live, considers my appearance to be of no great importance. If I wear jeans, a T-shirt, and tennis shoes he says, "I like this better than when you dress up. This is you." And he's completely serious. So I don't feel I have to put on, and primp, and fluff myself all the time. He's much more comfortable with the low-key life in general.

I definitely feel that I look better as I get older. I feel reasonably well-balanced in all areas of my life. I don't put as much emphasis on my appearance as I do on ability, intellect or personality. I have tried to find what works for me so appearance is no longer a consuming issue.

I see myself realistically as far as mirror image and self-image go. I stand in front of a mirror all day long during dance practice. I am still pretty concerned about the weight issue, so if my weight is okay, my self-image is realistic. But if my weight is up, I blow it out of proportion in my mind and then I panic.

For the most part, I am happy with the person I am today. However, I feel much more comfortable performing on stage in front of strangers than I do walking into a room full of people I don't know. I would love to feel more comfortable conversing easily with strangers. I would also like my dance image to have less influence over how I feel about myself.

For example, if I perform well on the night of a benefit performance, then I feel I deserve to attend the dinner dance, and I can push myself to be social because I feel worthy. It's a sick mentality, one that is pretty common among dancers. I would like to develop more separation between who I am and what I do.

The performance aspect of dance is extremely intense. If it's good, you feel wonderful about yourself, at least as good as your last performance. But if it's bad, it is very difficult to draw on your true self as unrelated to dance. You ride high on your performance and not on your personal esteem. A performance—two hours of intense physical contact with yourself, the other dancers, and with the audience—is very different than going to work in the corporate world or even just going to studio rehearsals every day. When we are on the road touring and performing constantly, I find it hard to separate who I am from what I do as a dancer. When we are in our home base for several months and I can see other friends and get involved in other projects and activities, I feel more well-rounded.

It's hard to say how I'll handle the aging process from this vantage point. If something becomes horrendous, I'll have it fixed, but otherwise I'll just deal with it. It doesn't scare me. Getting older makes me feel less influenced by the fashion magazine images. I hope that, as I age, I become more spiritual and introspective and leave behind the quest for success and competition. I hope I am passing into a new phase of life. I have had success in my career, and I have pretty much conquered my weight and metabolism problems, so I feel much more in control of myself and my accomplishments. It seems natural for looks to take a back seat to accomplishments in terms of who I am.

Several years ago, our whole dance company did an outdoor photo shoot. The crowd that gathered—thinking we were professional models— was in awe of us, our clothes, and our makeup. That was an interesting experience to me because I don't think of myself as model material, much less worthy of all the attention and photographic hoopla focused solely on appearance. I feel worthy of attention when I dance, but not for a photo shoot; the photo shoot experience didn't elevate me to model status in my mind, but the spectators didn't seem to differentiate.

I wonder how I would feel about myself if I hadn't had dancing and this constant weight problem on my hands all the time. I used to wish I had not gotten into this field so I could be "normal," but I probably would have found something else to worry about.

Thank heavens there is more flexibility in the fashion industry these days! There are so many more avenues to take now, not just one look. There used to be such a standardized or rigid way to look; now it's more acceptable to be different. And women themselves are becoming much more confident in having a style that may not necessarily be someone else's style. You see incredible diversity of appearance these days.

S A N D Y, 54:

aerobics instructor

I was a chubby little girl, constantly teased by my older sister that I was doomed to wear Chubbette clothes. However, by age 10 I was extremely thin—so thin that everyone's image of the chubby little girl disappeared. My sister, my brother, and I were all very skinny kids. "Thin" has always been my image of myself up until last year. Now at 54 years of age, I am filling out and getting more womanly.

In those early years, the worst thing was to be chubby; our society thinks thin is more acceptable than fat. I have always enjoyed being thin, and having people compliment me. Luckily, I didn't have to work at it—I was a chubby, full-faced, cute little kid and then suddenly I became very thin.

My parents always said good things and, in their own way, did the right thing. They weren't aware; they weren't tuned in to the psychology of their children. They were simply middle-class, hard-working people who were proud of their kids, and gave all three of us good feelings about ourselves. Even when I was chubby my mother and father thought I was adorable.

Unlike my weight, my personality has always been the same—outgoing and very talkative. I talked incessantly from the day I started talking, and I always had trouble in school because of it. I was constantly asked to leave the classroom because I loved to talk and laugh. I was happy-go-lucky, a little bit of the clown; I made everybody laugh. My family loved the fact that I was so funny. The teachers always liked me, too, because I was a good student, but they would send letters home to my mother saying, "Please explain to Sandy that she can't talk in school all the time." I've matured a little bit. Not a whole lot.

Physically, as a kid I was really cute. Then, as I got older, my nose grew faster than my face, so I had to contend with that in junior high and high school. I had my nose done when I was a senior in high school and that was a transformation in my self-image. The kids I went to school with didn't see the remodeling as anything unusual—it was a fairly common thing when I was growing up. I hate to say it was fashionable because we weren't in an economic group where everybody had a lot of money to have their nose done. But for the girls who needed it, and for a couple of the boys, it was very acceptable.

These operations were usually scheduled around Christmas and spring break because there was some time to recuperate. So after these holidays, some kids would come back looking a little different. People would say, "Oh, you look cute! Did you change your hair?" It wasn't treated as a big deal. But it was a big deal for the individual. It definitely changed the way I felt about myself; my self-image turned around. I never saw the surgery as the answer to other problems, though. For me it was pretty simple: get rid of this nose, I'll be a lot happier. I didn't have underlying complexes. I knew I was cute even with that nose. It was to make me happier, and to have the looks for professional dancing and photography work.

I have always had confidence. I went to dancing school and took ballet, modern dance, and jazz. Everyone knew I was a good dancer, and that set me apart from the rest of the kids, made me special and different. My talent always gave me confidence, but after having my nose done, I really felt good about myself. It balanced everything for me, gave me a lot of self-confidence. Maybe too much! I have always had very positive friends and I certainly had my share of positive reinforcement.

If a positive work experience and people's perception of you in the workplace is important to your self-esteem, then I have had the most positive experience a person could have. I have been teaching exercise classes for more than twenty years, and have developed a rapport with everyone in my class. Through the years I've met and become friendly with so many women. I can walk into class feeling lousy, but class is "show time" because everybody is so supportive. That support convinced me I had a lot more to offer than I realized.

When I first started teaching, I felt I was a fake; somebody was going to find me out. I was sure that I wasn't as good as people said, that I wasn't teaching correctly, and that I wasn't cutting it. Then other people started saying, "I heard about you! I want to be in your class." I lasted more than twenty years, so I am sure I wasn't a fake. And I had that reinforcement every single day. You don't often get that in a job.

So it's an incredible way to go to work every day. My working experience has given me self-confidence beyond anything I could have developed on my own. I am really indebted to the people who got me started teaching dance and exercise because it helped create the confident and outgoing person I am today. It carried over into raising my children, too; I was always confident of what I said to my kids. That confidence has really helped me to develop. Some people may say it's obnoxious, some say it's great, but it's certainly given me a wonderful feeling about myself. I am getting into real estate at this point in my life, which is a hard thing to do. I just felt I could do it. And everybody said, "You'll be great, do it!"

I married young, and although my husband took me away from professional dancing, he actually saved me from a lot of heartache in the world of professional dance. Some people are performers and some are teachers, and I have found that I am a teacher. I was so fortunate to find an outlet that was perfect for me; I was meant to do what I am doing.

So much of appearance is your attitude about yourself and what you do. It definitely shows in your face, your expression. I certainly didn't have these little lines a few years back, but it's part of the aging process. I probably looked better about ten years ago—at my best, really, in my mid-40s. I feel I'm going downhill, showing my age, but doing it fairly well.

Certainly, there is a gap of some kind between my mirror image and self-image; I don't see in the mirror what my friends see; I am hard on myself. I see these lines, and I wonder when they happened! If I see myself in a photo or video, I am never that pleased anymore. Everybody says I look great, but I don't see that myself. I see that in my mind's eye, but when I look in the mirror I am not that pleased anymore.

Although as a kid I went to dancing school, I was not as active or athletic as I am at this age. Now I am active in all kinds of sports. And I've added another level of accomplishment with athletics, because I married a man who is very athletic. I am not a fabulous athlete but I'm coordinated enough to learn and enjoy tennis, skiing, biking, and walking.

All this athletic activity in addition to my regular workouts in class has given me a tremendous amount of energy. Over the years I've increased my exercise capacity; the energy level is just there and I can accomplish a great deal without tiring. So I never thought I'd have a problem with the aging process. With my personality, I didn't think I'd notice menopause physically or mentally. But my body has changed; things are happening to me that I didn't expect. I've been very active with exercise and athletics, but I have no control over skin tone and texture. It has to do with genes and hormones and it's going to happen. I find that very hard to cope with.

And my figure has changed in the past two years; I'm not that skinny person anymore. My mother says I never looked better. I see her twice a year, and lately, at every visit I am a couple of pounds heavier. I feel uncomfortable, but she says, "Oh, no, you're not skinny anymore." For years my dad worried that if I got sick, I wouldn't recuperate, and then who would take care of my children? They just couldn't believe I was so thin even at 40 years old.

My husband says I am becoming more curvy, more womanly, and at this age I should have a little more meat on me. But I am having trouble dealing with it. This is the heaviest I have ever been. People still see me as cute and little, but I don't see myself that way any more. I think I am heavy, and in my head I am aging.

Shortly after retiring from my twenty-plus years as an aerobics instructor, I realized I had to suit up in my official exercise outfit to do my normal workout routine with focus. I needed my leotard, leggings, and headband for reinforcement. I found that if I just threw on sweatpants and a T-shirt, I fooled around and did a half-spirited routine. No uniform, no focus!

S H A N N O N, 24:
administrative assistant

My mom had a lot to do with my earliest memories of my appearance as a child. I was the baby, the only girl in the family, and she dressed me up in adorable outfits. She was grateful for a girl after three boys, the eldest of which was ten years older than I. For a while she had fun shopping for me and dressing me, but when my parents divorced we no longer had much money. I still have the dress I got for my third birthday—purple with little lace trim. It's really sweet. I also saved a darling sailor dress; Mom loved the sailor look.

In second grade I had long straight blonde hair, which I usually had cut at a good hair salon. But one time the hairdresser cut my hair really short, about chin length. It probably looked cute, but I was mortified. I never wore my hair short again until I got much older.

I felt positive about the way I looked. I never felt like a great beauty, but as the baby girl of the family, I got positive reinforcement and attention. Because I was only 6 months old when my father left and because my brothers took good care of me, I was sheltered from the divorce stuff. My mother dated a lot and then ended up marrying a very nice man. However, my dad was in and out of the picture, which was hard on my brothers. I don't remember it being so bad on me, but it was terrible on them. As teenagers, my oldest brother ran away and my middle brother, Joe, who often took care of me, had a nervous breakdown.

I thought I was pretty sheltered and I always felt loved, but there was still a lot of stress. I had many different babysitters, which was unnerving. Sometimes the lady who lived in the upstairs duplex babysat for me while caring for her own six kids. Her husband was so mean; he'd make those kids stand in the corner and eat. When I learned to write my name, I carved it into their coffee table in block letters: SHANNON.

I was always spoiled—not with material things but with attention. My mother, grandfather, and brothers all encouraged me in the special little girl role. My grandfather was a really dear person who loved girls.

Everyone said I was always so good; maybe I was too afraid to misbehave. But if I never misbehaved or was bratty, I never did boy things, either. I never played with my brothers or participated in their sports and they never encouraged me in that way. Like my real dad, my brothers have very traditional views of women, even if they appear to be liberal.

I was self-conscious and not very competitive. I had all kinds of dancing and ice-skating lessons and did well in sprinting, which is an individual effort, but I never did team things. To this day, team sports like softball make me cringe. My husband, Brian, says I'm uncoordinated, but the truth is I never played any sports and now I don't feel comfortable trying to learn.

In spite of the fact that I was always very girlish, I did well in the traditional boys' academic subjects like science and math. I grew up in Milwaukee and went to public school there, in a citywide magnet system of college-prep schools. I have always felt more sure of myself intellectually than physically. I never felt badly about the way I looked; I just never felt pretty enough or thin enough. I would have liked to be prettier. I've always wanted to be more fashionable looking, but I made a conscious trade-off to pursue intellectual things. Even now I feel I am not thin enough. Thin was really a big deal for us in school. My best friend, Sheila—who was always so thin—and I were both anorexic for a while. But I have always been very practical and I just got myself out of it. I suppose those appearance-related feelings held me back a bit, but I've always felt I got along well with people. I never had trouble meeting boys; I always had boyfriends. I was outgoing and assertive. I have a nice personality. Those things were trade-offs for not being the class beauty. Of course, I didn't want to be Miss Personality; I wanted to be Miss Legs.

I was always lucky to have good skin. That was THE BIG PLUS all those years. My hair was always a big positive, too. Now, however, my natural pale blonde hair is looking washed out. Why is it that hair is such a big thing? Even people with great hair hate it for some reason. Is there a woman alive who doesn't hate her hair?

Our school was very cliquish, as most are, with groups of perfect preppy girls with perfect hair who were very intimidating. They made me feel uncomfortable. Although I never belonged to a clique, I got along well with most people and pursued my own things in school. I was never really "in" but never really "out."

But then there was the clothes thing. The preppy crowd had their typical outfits, perfectly pressed and perfectly layered. They never looked stupid or bulky. There were also people who were really cool and more avant-garde—not quite punk, but leaning in that direction. They always dressed in black, which was pretty intense at age 15, but back then I thought it was cool. The lead singer of the Violent Femmes rock group went to our high school. Monkish to the extreme, he came to class every day in his bathrobe. I dressed conservatively, wearing a lot of men's big baggy shirts. I didn't have the nerve to be avant-garde in black lipstick and a bathrobe. Somebody actually commented that I always looked so straight and conservative, which wasn't the real me, but staying in the middle of the road style-wise was the best way to get along.

My looks were never a deterrent to anything I wanted to do or be, but there was one particular boy I liked for years whom I didn't get to date. He went with a girl who was tall and thin and put together, but she had a real nothing personality. She was perfectly blah. That made me feel terrible. She always looked as if a clerk at The Limited store had dressed her, with no creativity of her own. It was so depressing. She was pretty and thin and broad-shouldered and great looking and very aloof. I did go after him and we became very good friends, but I wasn't his type, obviously.

I am still learning to love myself the way I am. I would still like to be thinner. I'm not obsessed with my weight, but if I could be thinner it would make up for my nose, which I have always hated. I'm still only 24, so I've got many years to work on all this. I feel good enough about myself and my appearance.

My father was and still is obsessed with women. My mother said he always cheated on her. He kept an apartment so he could "go to the office" on Saturday mornings. When I asked her why she put up with him, she said she was wimpy then but not anymore. Leaving my mother with three young boys and a baby girl, my dad ran off to Australia with a woman named Roma. He wasn't around much when I was growing up, so there isn't much of a tie between us. I see him every so often. I feel angry about him.

A couple of years ago he took my brother Mike, and my husband-to-be, Brian, and me out to dinner. I had just started dating Brian at the time, so it was pretty embarrassing. Now that dad is older and doesn't have as much money, he is a stereotypical '60s playboy: open shirt, gold chains, flirtatious with waitresses. He's so old and pathetic that his act just doesn't work anymore. He flirted with the waitress and annoyed her so badly that I felt sorry for her. But when he asked for a hot towel at the end of the dinner in that casual restaurant, the waitress brought him a HandyWipe, which I thought was very creative! He insisted, "Honey, get a towel and run it under the hot water faucet." She looked enraged, walked away, and never brought the towel. Minutes later, when she came back with our coffee, his cup was filled to the brim. She slammed it down on the table, spilled coffee everywhere, and then walked away. She was so cool. But seeing it through Brian's eyes was horrible, especially so early in our relationship.

Dad is three times divorced now—the last two wives left him—and all he talked about was his latest girlfriend. His conversations were always obnoxious. He talked about women constantly, even in front of me. He talked about women's breasts, and about women he had slept with, and I'm sure he talked like that to my mother while they were married. It was so sick. It could have really warped my brothers and me.

Jenny Jones, the talk show host, tells a story about her father who sounds just like mine. Her father made an enormous issue about breasts the whole time she was growing up. Her breasts were never big enough and he laid that on her to the point that she eventually had breast implants. She has had them replaced about five times because of all the problems and finally had them removed. That kind of behavior by your father can really mess you up!

My two older brothers have very smart, sharp wives. Mike, however, married a woman more like my mother had been, and Mike runs the show. He's decent about it but he still bosses her around. Last time they came to visit, his wife wanted to get some opaque pantyhose, so we all went shopping and spent 20 minutes in the hosiery department while Mike decided on the pantyhose. When he tried to buy her some thigh-highs, I couldn't believe it. I said, "Real women don't wear those, they're for hookers. Don't let him do that to you, Mandy!" I am a lot more independent than Mandy. If Brian ever tried to tell me which pantyhose to buy, the locks would be changed and he'd be lucky if I set his suitcase out! My other two brothers try to tell their wives what to do, but their wives don't let them get away with it.

I went to college at the University of Wisconsin-Milwaukee. I decided to stay in town even though most of my high school friends were going to Madison. I moved out and lived away from home but I wasn't ready to leave the city. As I say, my brothers did a lot for me while keeping me tied to them throughout my college years as the babysitter for their kids. I probably stayed in Milwaukee for stupid reasons: a nice school, a lovely big-city campus right on the lake, a free-for-all atmosphere, and I had just met Brian. The campus was pretty diverse with a lot of older students and part-timers. I did well and was happy there, but it was dumb because my reasoning wasn't sound and I could have gone to a better school. I was only 18 and shouldn't have stayed for those reasons. Although I'm not sorry, I could have done it differently if I hadn't felt that I was indebted to my brothers and required to be well-behaved, considerate of everyone in the family, and academically responsible.

I majored in English after trying a boring business major. Because I was good in English and math, my brother tried to lure me into engineering, but that surely wasn't it. I tried English secondary education but I didn't really want to teach, so I finally ended up a basic English major. That was a relief for the rest of my school years, but now I have to balance it with the practical in real life. I don't feel I have to make a million before I'm 30, but I am creative and would like to use my abilities.

When I look at what happens within other families, I feel I have pretty solid self-esteem. From childhood on, I was always told that I was smart and could accomplish things. However, emotionally I still have a hard time doing things that might displease other people. It could be a little thing, like giving in on a choice of movies, or a big thing like a choice of schools. I am finally beginning to deal with the fact that I don't always have to please everybody. Sometimes it's easier to please than to deal with the hassles of doing what I want, but I am working on it.

I have the confidence to do almost anything, but I am not sure what it is that I want to do anymore. I got off the track. I graduated and didn't have a job, so I moved up to northern Wisconsin with Brian and worked while he went to graduate school. Then neither of us had anything specific to do, so we came to Chicago and worked with Brian's brother-in-law. When my brother Joe and his wife moved to LaCrosse, they were very disappointed that Brian and I had just moved to Chicago. They would have liked us to stay in Wisconsin so I could take care of their disabled child.

Some people can do something they don't particularly like all their lives. That's often a drawback of being a man because men get stuck doing things they don't want to do. Brian's dad was an engineer who hated engineering and who never wanted Brian to go into that field. So when Brian changed his major from engineering to accounting I said, "Why accounting? Why not meteorology?" He's such a weather freak; he loves to follow the weather. He'd be so cute for TV weather casting. But he wouldn't do it. Accounting was stable and professional. He worried that he'd disappoint his grandpa because he didn't go into engineering. The pressure is a family thing for him, too. Brian is currently working for a real estate company and doing well, but because he's not an Arthur Anderson CPA, the family cannot fathom what he does. It's so bizarre. We are both caught up in pleasing our family.

My parents' divorce was a terrible hardship on all of us. Dad's mother was just horrible and wouldn't have anything to do with us after the divorce. Personally, I'm glad Dad wasn't around. When my mom remarried, she chose a very nice, easy-going Mr. Milquetoast who was 15 years her senior and had grown kids. She probably did that on purpose. I was the only one still at home for the most part. They've had problems—he's content at home, she's still going strong; he's quiet, she is more social—but for me it was a fairly positive experience. I was lucky.

SHEILA, 50:
management consultant

One of my first memories as a little girl was of playing dress-up, my favorite pastime. Seeing myself looking gorgeous with high heels and Mother's makeup was fun stuff, a very positive experience for me.

As a youngster, most of the messages I remember being delivered by my mother were negative ones: how thin I was, how sallow my complexion was, the bags under my eyes. If I didn't get adequate sleep, the dark circles (from Dad's side of the family) would deepen. And my mother would be sure to remind me.

My mother was very controlling about my appearance and my style of dress. She allowed me very little choice in styling my hair and in choosing my clothes. I started doing my own hair in about fifth or sixth grade, when my mother began to rely on me to get my kid brothers up and all three of us off to school while she slept. So in my grammar school pictures, my hair was tragic! But what can you do at age 10 or 11? You don't really know how to work with your hair; you are just learning.

And then there was the Red Coat Incident when I was 10 years old. We had to buy my winter coat for that school year. I had my eye on a navy blue coat, but my mother picked out a red boy-coat with brass buttons. I thought it was very flashy and attention-getting. I disliked it tremendously. And it was at least three sizes too big for me because I was expected to get three years' wear out of such an expensive garment. Of course I lost the battle—and that theme continued until I left home at 18.

During preadolescence and all the way through high school, I felt that I was not okay: I didn't have a pug nose, wasn't blonde, didn't have big breasts—or breasts of any kind. I was still geeky, with a mouth full of teeth and no discernible development. In seventh and eighth grade, I distinctly remember stuffing my still unnecessary bra with nylons or Kleenex in order to feel that I had arrived.

I have lots of memories of the struggle to control my self-image and appearance even though I remained under the influence of my mother. My father regarded me as Daddy's little girl. I'm his only daughter, so I got a lot of validating messages from him although he was often absent. But he certainly didn't play a role in choosing my clothes, or how I wore my hair, or whether I wore makeup. That's where Mom jumped in. And stayed in. For special occasions she took me to the bathroom and dusted my cheeks with rouge to give me needed color. She was really saying, "You are not okay the way you look," but the "con" was to be like Mom with a little makeup.

My major act of rebellion against my mother was in eighth grade. I had dark auburn hair and was very hirsute, which I found totally repugnant. So I broke the rules and shaved my very hairy legs. It was my emancipation from her strings. And what could she do about it? I was very proud of myself.

For Easter of that year, my mother gave me money to buy shoes to go with the outfit she had picked out for me. Thank God she couldn't buy the shoes on her own. Guess what I bought? Three-inch navy blue spike heels! In 1956. In eighth grade. My mother almost died but she did not make me return the shoes. She was just as caught up in my maturation as I was. When I brought those shoes out to show my father, he made me put them on and practice walking. It was hilarious! And he went on and on about a woman not wearing high heels unless she knows how to walk and carry herself properly. That was his contribution to my appearance.

I was a slow grower-upper: slow to start wearing makeup, tweezing my very heavy eyebrows, and manicuring my nails. My only high school chums were girls. I was sexually very immature and naïve; I dated very little. I went to the senior prom on a last-minute fix-up deal. My senior high school picture was pretty standard: classic page-boy hairdo with the barrette, very little makeup. A very natural kid. I wanted long hair in a ponytail, the rage, but my hair wasn't long enough.

The big fashion trend at my high school was Pendleton skirts and matching sweaters. But they were out of my reach, along with the one-pearl-on-the-gold-chain necklace, and the gold circle pin. I worked part-time and bought a few clothes, but I kept my desires pretty well under wraps. It was kind of sad.

At the University of Iowa, I changed overnight, like a butterfly literally coming out of my cocoon. I went through Rush Week, pledged a house, and went to the pledge dance. All the fraternities and sororities attended this big dance, which was my first social event at college. And I'll be damned—I never sat down! One guy after another asked me to dance! And when I left that dance, I had dates with different guys for every day of the week, for the next three weeks straight. And I was on my own! That was the best part.

Thus began my college career. I suddenly got messages that men and women found me attractive. I dated! I had the most unbelievable social life during college. I played hard. And I worked very hard. I had the best of everything. I got good grades and had a great social life; it was just a wonderful time for me. And I was nominated for queen of this, and court of that, and sweetheart of this or that fraternity.

In my first two months at college, I changed my whole style: wrap-around wool skirts with cardigans, knee socks, tennis shoes (white Keds, the dirtier the better) and, of course, the trench coat. And when I came home at Thanksgiving, my parents just looked at me. "My God, who is this? She looks so different." But they liked what they saw! I got a lot of reinforcement. From then on, my looks and self-image were quite positive. I felt very good about the way I looked and presented myself. I felt very confident about my style.

Then the college community had a beauty contest, the Miss Safe Boating of Iowa pageant. One hundred bucks for the winner. My girlfriends put me up for it. I had worked on my tan and went decked out in my white Lanz bathing suit with falsies in the top. Got second place and won fifty bucks! And a lot of laughs! First runner-up for Miss Safe Boating of Iowa.

I was asked to model—fashion show modeling, photo modeling for the school newspaper. Suddenly I was getting all kinds of messages that my appearance was okay, even without a big chest, or pug nose, or blonde hair.

During my senior year of college, I remember consciously making the decision to buy clothes that I could wear as a single career woman. I stopped buying college clothes, and started building a wardrobe for the workplace. By the time I graduated and moved East, I understood that appearance—what you wear, how you accessorize, and how you do your face and hair—can make you look like Betty Co-ed, a beatnik, or a businesswoman. I revealed all those different aspects of myself, depending on how I merchandised myself, and was very comfortable with it emotionally. No problem whatsoever. What a terrific realization!

As a single career woman and then a young married, I became even more sophisticated. I wore my hair pulled straight back in a chignon at the nape of my neck. I modeled in more charity events. In my 30s, despite two 50-pound pregnancies and two 9-pound babies, I retained my figure. I started paying more attention to my shape, although I didn't do anything to help it.

When I was 35 years old, I went to a professional training course related to my business. The course got into a lot of personal growth issues and was very intense. I had worked very hard to integrate the material, questioning and interacting with both my instructor and fellow trainees. On the afternoon of the last day, the instructor set up a structured experience to help the group separate from the event and plan for the future. The exercise involved one-on-one feedback between rotating pairs, each person sharing his or her experience of the other—positive or negative, any kind of feedback. When it was over, I broke down in tears and sobbed uncontrollably.

Virtually without exception, the feedback I got was negative! The women said things like, "You threaten me because you are so beautiful, or because you dress so beautifully. I'm jealous of you." The men said, "I'm very attracted to you sexually. I'm very threatened by you as a powerful woman." Everything had to do with my physical appearance and nothing was about my intellect! It tore me apart! And for the first time in my life, despite all my experiences up to that point, I realized how many people saw me solely in terms of appearance.

I don't look at myself in every window and mirror; my energies go elsewhere. So to go through a weeklong educational event and have no one see the intellectual or human part of me was very upsetting. The group saw only my appearance, my style, my sexuality, and translated them into negative fear and jealousy. But it ultimately became a great experience, because it taught me that, especially in business, I had to be very careful about the messages I sent women as well as men. I had to work very hard with women so that they would not be intimidated by me, and with men so that they would not be distracted by my appearance. It was a brutally painful experience for me, but it became a real asset.

My age is often underestimated by both men and women, particularly if I am in a dimly lit room. Even in the daylight, most people do not figure that I'm 50. Still I have struggled with my appearance this past year. My face has aged a lot due to enormous stress. I see wrinkling around my mouth. I know it's not just because I smoke. My mother has never smoked and she has the same patterns. The laugh lines and the wrinkles around the eyes and on the forehead don't bother me. It's just the general tone and the "purse strings"—those bother me. Since my early 40s, I have had a perfect streak of silver hair. My kids hate it and my mother says it ages me. So I've hit the bottle to cover up the gray. I don't know how long I want to keep doing it.

I have been addressing aging issues since my 30s, but at 50, it's a stretch to feel okay with my self-image. I can affirm myself by looking at other women my age and thinking, "I am blessed." But we live in a culture that honors youth and, no matter how gracefully I age, I'm not part of that anymore. It's not so much dissatisfaction with my looks as with the experiential changes as a result of our culture.

In my career, however, aging has actually been an asset. I'm in the management consulting business, and I have found that organizational executives feel much more comfortable with someone who has a few gray hairs, some wrinkles, and a little mileage, than with a younger person. Six years ago another consulting firm hired me to work on a European project. It couldn't send its young Ph.D.s, whose credibility had not yet been established, to work with senior executives. So age has been a real asset in my work.

I see myself in my mind's eye just as I am now. I know exactly how I look to others. I rarely wear makeup unless I'm seeing clients. And I'm comfortable; I don't need makeup to do things in the neighborhood.

I would say that my appearance ranks equally with my intellect, achievements, and personality. Whatever successes I have had are a product of both my ability and my appearance. I would hate to have a pathetic personality. I would hate to be ugly. I consider my appearance to be a tremendous asset, not just because of my style, or the way I look or dress, but because of what I learned in that seminar fifteen years ago.

I learned that although people like to be around other attractive people, I have an obligation to help them get through any barriers. In order to help people get past strong feelings of threat, jealousy, intimidation, or fear—feelings that have been incited by me—I have to reveal my vulnerabilities and my humanness to them, because they can't see those qualities for themselves. Those who are blessed with a pleasing appearance need to be aware of how they may affect others, especially if they want to help people get into the relationship on a level where it's not how-you-look versus how-I-look, or what-you-have versus what-I-have. Those ideas get in the way of doing business, of sharing a friendship, of loving each other.

Feedback about how we look and how we act is a basic requirement if we are going to change and grow. The sad thing is that a lot of us don't invite the feedback or we reject it out of hand, because we would have to change, and that's scary. The real leap of faith is that we need to listen to what other people tell us, verbally and nonverbally, about how they see and experience us. And we need to seriously consider that feedback, because maybe we need to change something.

It's important to pay attention to your intellectual development, your career, your family, and your social life. Appearance should not be ignored, but it should not be given the obscene amount of attention that Madison Avenue and our culture give it. That's a waste. There are more important things to worry about. Plastic surgery is one way people cope with our culture, but you really have to learn to cope with yourself first.

S H E L L E Y, 30:
labor and delivery nurse

My earliest memory of myself is as a 4-year-old when I walked by a mirror and saw myself with a pixie hair cut and fire engine red hair. It was very orange-red and definitely made me stand out. By the time I was 8 or 9 years old other kids figured out I was different and started saying things like, "You're odd, you have red hair!"

I was the only redhead in my class at school—and the only redhead in my family. My father was one of twelve siblings, so I have sixty-some first cousins and seventy-some second cousins, and none of them has red hair. At family functions with mobs of people, I was the only one with red hair, which was attributed to a great-great grandfather. So I felt different, not negatively, just different.

My early elementary school years were pretty uneventful until my fifth-grade major growth spurt; then I grew really tall. I was a head, or a head and a half, above almost everyone else in school. By junior high, though, I wasn't as tall by comparison. The other girls had started to catch up to me, and then the boys had their big growth spurts. But during that whole time I was embarrassed to go to other kids' houses because I was so clumsy.

Throughout my gymnastics classes I never saw myself as heavy, just tall. However, by late high school and college, I also thought I was heavy. According to the charts I was average in weight, but 15 or 18 pounds heavier than I am now. In college I was in the ballet and modern dance group, and because I was the tallest, I thought I was the biggest. Tall and big was akin to fat. I was troubled by my weight.

During high school and early college, girls are supposed to put on weight as a natural part of the maturation process, but that fact gets lost in the whole physiology of menstruation, water weight, and breast and hip development. So girls are unaware of that fact and fight the necessary weight gain because they don't realize it's normal. Look at the eating disorders today at age 12 or earlier; misinformation allows girls to see themselves as fat and then starve to look good or feel good.

I don't remember my parents ever commenting on how I looked. I was affirmed for accomplishments and grades, but they never said, "You look good. That dress is nice. You've done your face nicely." There was only one negative comment on my looks. At my high school graduation party, my favorite uncle, Bill, was chatting with my father when I came into the room. My dad looked at me and said, "Why are you wearing eye makeup? You look so much better without any makeup!" I was really vulnerable, and on my special day Dad had said that in front of my favorite uncle. I know Dad didn't do it maliciously; his daughter was growing up and he liked her the way she was. But the only thing he had ever said made me feel bad. He could have said, "Here's my gorgeous, wonderful, smart daughter of whom I am so proud!"

I remember that incident distinctly, but I don't remember anything else that my parents ever said about my appearance. They didn't comment on my sister or brothers, either. They saw only our capabilities, or, perhaps, they didn't know they should comment positively on our appearance.

My clothes never fit, and all I ever wanted was something that was long enough for me. I wore boys' pants because they were longer, but I felt everyone knew they were boys' pants. Also, I remember testing colors on myself and saying "Mom, you can't buy me anything pink or mustard-colored." But my mom didn't take my suggestions and I had to wear those awful colors!

In high school, I didn't feel unattractive, but many people were more attractive than I—more developed, or cuter. I was the girl next door, and the guys were more interested in the beauty queens and the cheerleaders, or the basketball and volleyball stars. I played in the band and ran track where there was no built-in spectator group.

I was always an organizer in high school. I was the class president for a number of years and did theater, but never be-boppy things. Maybe those restrictions were self-imposed because I didn't feel confident or comfortable enough, or as cute as other girls. I was a leader—the farthest thing from any guy's mind. So did I push the men away because I was a leader, or did I assume leadership because I felt I couldn't attract dates? I honestly don't know.

I didn't date in high school, but I didn't miss out on much, either. A lot of us didn't date, but were always in big mixed groups. Our band was half men and half women and we all went out for pizza after a game. The theater crowd was like that too, with a big mix of people and wonderful parties, "heady" parties, with substance and enough conversation to solve all the world's problems. It was a good social life, safe and all-American. We were interested in real life issues and had no pretenses—and no gang problems.

I had a very nice adolescence insulated from the peer pressure of dating. Some of it was geographic—living four miles outside of town with no close neighbors, I hung out with my sister and my brothers. My parents were very active and involved with us in team sports. Every summer we had our own backyard softball team.

I loved to read and study and I got good grades. Within the family I was affirmed for accomplishments when no one else was. My sister, who is a year older and learning disabled, took special education classes and was slower but had her own achievements. I felt guilty being recognized by my parents for an A, because it was a far greater achievement for my sister to get a B. Yet I was recognized for things when my sister wasn't. That was a tough issue to deal with; I didn't want to be affirmed disproportionately to my sister and brothers. During my college years I wanted to break family ties and simultaneously tell my parents these things, explaining my guilt. I tried to make my mother aware by saying, "I want you to say good things about the others, and not just about me," but my mother didn't understand or register anything. I wasn't pressured to succeed, but I felt as if I had to fill the firstborn's shoes by default. I didn't need to succeed for my parents—I just liked to succeed. At some point, though, I said, "I don't want this sole affirmation."

My parents are very open, honest people and wouldn't hurt anyone. They never went to college, aren't into current pop psychology, and don't realize the importance of "strokes." But we turned out fine, I guess. I don't feel as if I have any big gaps. My parents struggled to raise us with whatever tools they had. Group participation: "Let's get out there and play games and go camping. Do things as a family." That was wonderful. That's something a lot of kids never have.

Because of my feelings about being singled out by my parents, I volunteered for the Peace Corps when I graduated from college. I wanted to be on my own and make it on my own, for myself and not for my parents' expectations. I wanted to go away to see if I could survive and develop my personal strengths and inner qualities.

I was sent to a small village in Africa as a teacher. Africa was a very, very positive experience. I didn't have to worry about how I looked in relation to other whites. I wasn't different from people of my own race; I was different from people of a different race. I was different because I had white skin, and straight hair. It wasn't about fitting a certain aesthetic mold.

I explored who I was, what I felt good wearing, what fabrics and colors I felt comfortable in. I found myself very connected to cotton fabrics and earthy colors in Africa. I could tell the fundi, the maker of clothes, that I wanted this color or that style. Or that I wanted to use her sewing machine to make such and such. It was tough coming back to the United States. I was gone from '84 to '86, when everyone did this seasonal color thing. And when I came back, people would say, "That's an interesting color! What season are you?" Well, I had discovered my own colors in my own way. It was for me, and also of me; no one told me what to wear.

Sometimes here in the States I succumb to outside pressure from the enormous choices available, and don't wear the things I'm most comfortable in. Many of my favorite things are muted in color, or undefined in shape or style. I am conscious that I don't dress as sharply as others do, but it often bothers others if I wear my favorite natural things. Because I am conscious of pleasing others, I often tone down my clothing, or add a necklace. I realize that I am sacrificing some of myself, but if I think the other person will feel more comfortable, that's important to me, too. I guess it's a social tool, just like conversational ability.

I have never worked in jobs where appearances are an issue. As a teacher and a nurse, you don't worry about how you look because you are a necessity. But I do put much thought into dressing for the occasion. For instance, I wouldn't teach small children dressed in a black suit, it's too authoritarian, intimidating, and unapproachable. I consciously adapt to the needs of the audience. When I came back from Africa I got another degree; I am a labor and delivery nurse now, and wear scrubs at work. So there you are: green color, no style. I never have to worry about what to wear!

While teaching in Africa, I never thought about those things. I wore comfortable boxy blouses and loose skirts all the time. Jeans were taboo—they connoted "loose woman," the "wenchy" kind from American movies. The Peace Corps clothing guidelines said to cover up our body: high necklines, long skirts. Look approachable and comfortable to the Africans. Promote the good American image.

I met my husband, Paul, in Africa. He was finishing medical school with an international Third World public health component at the mission hospital in my village. I met him, one Sunday, on the road outside the village. He waved and called me masungu, which is like "honky." All the little kids had been calling him that, and he thought it meant "hi" or "how are you doing?"

During my stay in Africa, my only mirror was four inches by six inches, so all I saw was my nose! My nose had been broken in a childhood softball game and, having healed incorrectly, had a pronounced bone projection. I had always wanted to get the bone aligned or reshaped. After we were married, Paul did a residency rotation through plastic surgery. The plastic surgeon operated on my nose and Paul assisted. They shaved the bone down nicely. It's subtle. I still think I have a big nose, but it's more graceful. So I have done something about my looks, and I feel better about myself. At the same time, I can't see myself doing any other kinds of cosmetic surgery. On a small scale, my nose was a social inhibition: I thought people saw me as tall, red-haired and large-beaked, so I sat back and waited for social things to happen. I never asked a guy out because I didn't feel I measured up. I have often heard women say that glasses made them feel that way. Interestingly for me, glasses hid my nose! I wear my contact lenses when we go out socially, but I wear my glasses more often, as camouflage.

I always had a very flat stomach but now I have this little cushiony area—a post-childbirth paunch. I do tons of situps and try to breathe just right to develop the muscle correctly, but I still have this belly. It sounds crazy and I try not to focus on it. Guys don't have this focus; they don't think about it. It's definitely a gender thing. Women are caught up in this stuff.

Acne has become a big issue for me these days. I never had acne as a teen, but now, in my 30s I have an acne problem. And I am so focused on it. We socialize with other physicians and their wives—very affluent and educated people—and here I am with this thing on my face! It's awful. I see other people with an outbreak, and I don't really notice it or let it make a difference in the way I feel about them. But I don't feel that same generosity toward myself or give myself credit for other features and attributes and abilities that outweigh a facial blemish. This acne can really set the tone for the way I feel about myself: I get obsessed about it and

I don't want to be around people. How sad to give in to this self-imposed negative feeling about myself!

There are days when I just don't feel good about myself and I wonder why Paul married me. I certainly do not have his caliber of looks. I'm the girl next door, with the slim, trim, athletic build and the all-American looks. Thank God the Marilyn Monroe look isn't in anymore!

In ranking my attributes, I would rank my personality highest: I think I have a funny personality and am fun to be around. Further on down the list would be my physical characteristics. And the words I choose to describe myself are strong, caring, nurturing—words that aren't tied to physical appearance. I'm not unattractive, just a pretty average person. However, I am not striving toward physical beauty as I get older. I am actually getting more comfortable with my looks. Eventually you get past looks. At least I hope so—that's certainly the goal.

My self-image is balanced with others' perceptions of me now. I see myself pretty much the way I think I am perceived. I focus more on personality, abilities, and comfortable traits; I try not to focus on appearance. Maturation is a long process that comes with age and experience ultimately. Aging? Hey, let it happen! Feeling good about myself physically is more important. I simply want to maintain my weight and stay trim.

A big part of my personality is caretaking and resourcefulness because we didn't have a lot of money when I was growing up. There were no frills. I made my own clothes; I could never pay someone else to do it. My arms are exceptionally long, so as a kid, I always had to roll up my too-short sleeves. As a result of those youthful wardrobe problems, I am very conscious of buying "talls" and finding sleeves that are long enough to cover the lower third of my arm. This year Paul finally convinced me to buy a new coat. It's green and very classic and I feel great in it. I've always wanted a green coat. And I actually spent the $15 to have someone else let down the sleeves! Usually I do it myself. But I am treating myself this time.

FOOTNOTE: I am becoming more comfortable with my looks as I age—more accepting, coming into love of self. I realize it's all about soul and has nothing to do with externals. I think I always knew this, but was afraid to trust it.

I am a runner now. I started jogging post-partum—after my daughter was born nine and a half years ago. I just ran a two-man/woman marathon. Every day I run four to five miles—a gift of quiet and solitude and prayer and exercise I give myself.

Being apart from my husband, I see clearly how I let myself grow weaker in love of and contentment with myself over the years. The last lines of a poem—a work in progress—"my face, my dance, my song, they are me now."

STACY, 19
college student

When I was a child, my parents were always positive about me, but my brother called me dumb and ugly and fat and creepy. That took hold and I began to see myself that way—as fat, at least. I also ran into problems with four of the most popular girls in my grade school who started an against-Stacy campaign. I had stopped using my first name, Ann, and started using my middle name, Stacy; I had also cut and permed my hair in tight curls like "Annie." Those girls followed me around and took notes, making up things about me like, "Now she's picking her nose, now she's biting her nails." But I think they finally respected me because I am independent and not afraid to be different. They finally tapered off the harassment and stopped the game.

I didn't like my looks until I got my braces off on Valentine's Day of my junior year in high school. Then, when I got my first serious boyfriend, I was the most conceited person around for about six weeks. After that I settled down.

My girlfriends have been supportive for the most part. My best girl-friend has always told me how pretty I am. Even my bosses at the restaurant where I worked during the summer were very upset when I left to go to college. They said I was the prettiest waitress and that I brought in a lot of business. The men I've dated have always been complimentary, too. I have gotten most of my positive feelings about myself from the men I've dated. They have always been affirming. Even my brother is very positive these days. Now he threatens to kill me if I ever cut my hair, which I am currently wearing very long and straight.

For several years in high school, I wore really baggy clothes— four sizes too big—to cover up my weight. After losing some weight, I came into school one day in the right size jeans, and everyone really complimented me. That helped me see myself in a better light.

I never really dieted to lose the weight. A friend and I saw a TV movie about a single mom who was an exercise fanatic and a bulimic. My friend was studying ballet and was considered overweight, so we decided to try eating and purging, even though bulimia almost killed the movie character. I got into it because of my friend and did it when I was around her, but not at home where I ate regular meals. However, I was the one who got caught in the lavatory at school by one of the counsellors and taken to the guidance center. I simply couldn't have my parents find out. The counsellors promised not to tell my parents if I came to group sessions twice a week for a period of time. I don't think my mom ever found out. I told her I was working on a play. I always knew I wasn't hooked on bulimia, and even though I hadn't liked being overweight I also hid the weight loss under those baggy clothes. When I got caught purging, I just stopped.

I feel best about myself now; I wouldn't go back to even a year ago. I'm not totally pleased, but I'm content with my looks. I don't think of myself in physical terms as much as independent, accomplished, focused, aware of who I am and what I want.

I'm an elementary education major in college. I love kids; they're my hobby and my intended career. I've been babysitting since I was 10 and I would rather do that than go out with my friends in a group.

Right after I came home for the summer following my freshman year in college, my boyfriend's buddy had a college graduation party scheduled for their group. But when one of my favorite families called me to babysit that same night, I agreed because I'd missed being with kids so much. As it turned out, my boyfriend picked me up later and we went to the party after my job was finished. It worked out great.

I think my intellect and accomplishments are more developed than my self-image. Although other people seem to think highly of me, I still put myself down too much. It's one of the things my boyfriend complains about the most. My mom often reminds me about that, too. I'm working on it.

S YLVIE, 35:
bank executive

I don't have a clear recollection of my appearance as a child growing up in a small town in France, other than that people said I had big eyes. At the age of 5 I had freckles, which I didn't like, but my grandmother reassured me they were normal—there was nothing wrong with those little dots. My recollection of who I was had more to do with my personality than my looks at that point.

However, at age 14 I went to boarding school for three years where I immediately gained a tremendous amount of weight. That was a big problem because I had been taking ballet lessons for years and loved dancing. But at 14 my whole body changed to what I called my 19th-century body. I have the same kind of body as Renoir's models: big legs and a small torso.

I had always had a big appetite and my mother, who was not the most empathic woman in the world, said that if I continued eating like that, I would become the size of my obese grandmother. That was a meaningful threat because my grandmother was particularly big and fat even though she was relatively young.

I lost weight after that year, and once in a while the issue of fat legs would come up and irritate me, but it wasn't a major part of my formative years. My friends and I were more interested in our intellect; we didn't have to have our hair in a certain style or weigh a mere 100 pounds to feel appealing. Because I wasn't interested in boys, there was not a lot of pressure on me about appearance. In fact, my mother never bothered me about it although she constantly bugged my sister about her big nose—to the point where my sister had a nose job at age 24.

Mother used to say to me, "The only reason I married your father was because I got pregnant with you." Although that statement could have totally devastated me, my attitude was always, "It's not my fault!" If I hadn't been so matter-of-fact about it, I probably wouldn't have turned out the way I did. I became stronger, more independent, more forceful.

Appearance was secondary because I simply had to have a strong backbone to get through life.

Ballet and music were my escape from the family situation as well as my salvation: I could do and be whatever I fantasized and be absolutely happy. Dance provided a strong part of my identity, although I never considered it a career choice. It provided a satisfying and peaceful environment where I could be my own person. So, although I could have felt bad and put guilt on myself, I didn't and I don't know why. I never even thought about the negatives until many years later.

My parents and sibling really played a positive role in my self-image in spite of themselves. My sister and I had a tough relationship when we were growing up. I didn't care for her; she was jealous of me. But we did support each other because we were both caught in our unhappy family situation. My mother threw tantrums and threatened to commit suicide on a regular basis. She often went off in her car and pretended to kill herself. Whenever that happened my sister really freaked out, although I never did. Mother finally stopped that behavior when, as a teenager, I confronted her and told her to kill herself, instead of just talking about it. I was tired of her game!

As the eldest of the immediate cousins, I was regarded as responsible; mature for my age, I looked older than I was. Determined to do well on the very difficult exams which allowed me to both graduate from high school and enter the university, I was a serious student. My only diversion was ballet. I didn't date. I had a few select friends with whom I developed close relationships, but I was never part of a group that could influence me much. On the other hand, my sister tried desperately to fit into the wrong group. As a result, the social pressure was greater on her than it ever was on me.

In our family there was a tradition of education for girls. My parents, my aunt, and my cousins were all teachers. So there was no question that our brains came first. There was never any doubt that we would get the best education we could in terms of college and advanced studies. It would have been a catastrophe if we hadn't succeeded. In fact, the only time I got a cum laude instead of a magna cum laude on my exams, my mother said, "What happened?" in a tone of voice that was like doom.

Schooling was always my priority, and the discipline of studying was reinforced by my ballet and music practice. There was a lot of work involved. My ballet became a problem at boarding school, because I wanted to continue to take lessons and perform with the ballet school students. My parents negotiated a deal with the school whereby I was allowed to go out at night to perform but I had to maintain straight A's. And I couldn't fail because the school was making a major exception to its traditional policy. So on those nights that I was performing and didn't get back to the dorm until 11:00, I spent another couple of hours studying under the covers. I had to make sure I didn't fail because it meant too much to me.

I was really uncomfortable about becoming like my mother, who was very vain. Just 21 years older than me, she is frightened to death of getting old. She has always been that way. She is very proud of having had children very young because it was a compliment to her sexuality, her sexiness, her appeal. I always found that very uncouth. The one thing I didn't want to be was like her. So when I finished college, I emigrated to the United States where I completed a teaching assistantship in Ohio, earned my master's degree, and was awarded a Rotary scholarship in Minneapolis. I felt absolutely free of all kinds of things and I felt very good about everything, including the way I looked.

I recently celebrated my birthday and I don't mind admitting I am 35 and love every minute of it. I am not afraid of aging or losing my façade. I believe much of a woman's beauty comes from a healthy outlook on life, a positive attitude, and a good personality. And there are advantages to not being beautiful— you work harder on other things. And you don't have to worry about your looks so much. There is a lot of pressure from peers, parents, and society in general that I, frankly, never wanted to succumb to. The only thing that gets to me is a weight issue. If I start gaining too much weight and it's out of control, it bugs me because I've lost discipline more than anything else. I know I have close-set eyes and a big nose, but what am I going to do about it? Sometimes I have good hair days, and sometimes bad hair days, but I'm not going to freak out. In other ways I am stronger than that, and that's what matters to me.

Not that I wouldn't want to have the perfect body and a beautiful face, but if it isn't there in the first place or with a little bit of general maintenance, then that's fine. It's not what I look for in people, so I don't want people to look for that in me. When I was 16 I found in my mother's drawer an anonymous letter that someone in town had sent to her. She was into lots of civic activities, so I suppose some disgruntled committee member had written her this nasty letter. It described my mother as "so proud of her daughters—one with big legs and the other with a big nose!" I didn't like reading it but it was true to a certain degree; I couldn't pretend I had skinny legs. But my sister also saw that letter, which sent her into a big crisis. I didn't react like that. Somehow I divorced myself from it all.

Frankly, with this my first pregnancy, I have gained a lot of weight— more than I should have, especially in my thighs—and I got worried. It's one thing to be a little heavy, but I didn't want to look repulsive. My grandmother phobia returned in force. So I went to a nutritionist right away and found out what I was doing wrong. She put me back on the right track. If my metabolism makes me gain 60 pounds instead of 35, as long as I am eating right, there is nothing else I can do.

On a personal level, I'm probably the happiest I've ever been. When I was a young single woman living in Ohio and Minnesota, I had a great time doing whatever I wanted. I was free as a bird. But now I know where

I am going and what I want out of life. I know what my limitations are and, yes, I'm getting older but I'm also getting smarter. If you are healthy, maturing is great. Every day has pleasure in it. I feel the best I've ever felt. It's due to finding myself, doing what I want to be doing, being challenged.

My most positive image of myself is healthy and healthy-minded with a very positive outlook. I am upbeat, determined, and strong-minded. As a kid, I was always so strong that, even if I was sick, my parents never took it seriously: "Oh, Sylvie will be fine!" And they still treat me that way. Physically and mentally healthy is what I think I am about. I may do things to please other people, but I please myself first.

I don't think my looks were better at a younger age. Extra weight after childbirth may be a problem, but mental attitude at any age is key. Going through middle age, a divorce, problems in a marriage or with children, problems at work, can all contribute to feelings about your looks. I don't expect to stay looking young as I get older, but I don't expect my appearance to be an issue unless major health problems come along.

I think my intellect, personality, and achievement come first. My appearance is part of the package, but I definitely think my personality is the driving force. And I feel pretty good about myself, I must say, although there are always things to work on. I disassociate myself from people I don't care to be around and if I am this confident, I might be perceived as arrogant or way too sure of myself, which can be a drawback. So I hope I don't give that impression.

I am strong and I come across that way; however, it doesn't mean I'm not vulnerable, which surprises some people. But I don't think there is much of a gap between what I think of myself and what others think. I am pretty good at stepping out of myself and observing from a distance.

As far as the aging process goes, staying healthy is the main thing. I plan to deal with aging in a very different manner than my mother, who is so petrified of growing old. I haven't thought about it much yet, beyond the possibility of losing a friend or family member. I just want to take it in a very healthy manner and be appreciative of daily pleasures.

A friend was discussing with me her role as the fifth child and baby of the family, who was never allowed to be herself. She has always been amazed at my stories of how I have stepped out of myself. Because my childhood wasn't all that great, I have waited a long time to have my own children. I don't feel that raising children should be done lightly; people have to be really ready and able to step away from their old family issues to avoid repeating them. I avoid going back to France to visit because my parents, though they are still young, are in patterns that they will not change. And I can't do anything about it. If I start reacting to them, then I fall into the same patterns. I have to stay as distant from those patterns as possible.

POSTSCRIPT: During my second pregnancy, at age 38, I ate better and gained less. I still had an extra 15 pounds in all the wrong places, and it finally got to me. I have had a personal trainer for over a year, have lost 20 pounds, am stronger than ever and still nurse my toddler. At this stage I am really enjoying myself, my new career as a public relations consultant, my husband, my two children and my friends.

TRUDY, 47:
arts activist, fund-raiser

My first memories of myself as a child and of my mirror image are negative because I was born with one ear whose lobe, like a little teardrop, came down but wasn't attached to my cheek. As a child, I didn't want to be different from anyone else, so my earlobe bothered me and I always wanted it covered up. Those feelings led to insecurity as a small child.

In addition, I went to a German Lutheran parochial school with kids whom I perceived as different from me. Whether I knew the difference was economic or social, I can't say, but there was always a feeling of "them and me." And I always ended up hanging around with guys like Vernon, a sad-sack little fellow. He and I would play and "they" would play.

I never felt that I looked the same as the other kids, either. I remember looking at Beverly's skirt and realizing I didn't have one of those. At that time I hadn't formulated my own sense of taste (or wasn't allowed to), and couldn't make any "chooses" for myself. But I was aware that the things I had didn't fit in.

Talk about incidents in childhood that affect you! These memories are from kindergarten and are still very vivid. I feel now that children are often mean, and I felt then that they were mean to me. I remember crying a lot.

However, I could sing. And I could sing well enough that "they" asked me to sing in the Christmas program. But then that caused friction too. The Lutheran mothers didn't think I should take part in the program because my mother was Methodist. I thought she was a perfectly nice lady. But that stuff was all very symptomatic of the times.

Whatever faults my parents might have had, they contributed very positively to my self-image. They were very ecumenical people and I never heard them speak derogatorily about anyone. We lived in several different areas and they always encouraged me to go to whatever church I chose and thereby meet other children. Although I went to the Lutheran school, I also attended the Catholic Sunday school. And then later on I had lots of Jewish friends. It was fun to see who was out there; it allowed me to have a broader base and helped me acclimatize to the narrower viewpoint in school.

But then in sixth grade we moved far enough away so that I could not realistically go to that school anymore. I had to go to public school. Well, there is no question that the move enhanced my self-esteem because I was way ahead of the public school kids; my education at the Lutheran school had been very good. My advanced academics gave me the time to concentrate on a little social life and the chance to be a little competitive. And school was close to home, which allowed me more freedom in terms of who I was. That was my jumping off point to be much more popular, which is so important in those formative years.

So I ended up a grade school cheerleader and figured out that being at the head of things was not such a bad deal. I realized that I was motivated and had some organizational talent as well. Coincidentally, I was now singing competitively at my new school, and winning contests, though I had not had singing lessons. My folks were very positive about my talent. Plus, their backstage behavior was nice and solid. My younger brother, Randy, looked up to me in those years, too. All of that made me see myself very positively in the mirror.

By high school I was in pretty good shape: I was a class leader and involved in cheerleading, drama, and music. The tomboy part of me got interested in baseball and that allowed me to be really good friends with boys. Although there was less romance, there was some good feedback because I learned about boys' likes and interests and developed some real social graces about the male-female thing. Strangely enough, I didn't develop girlfriends until later. In high school, sleep-overs and heart-to-heart conversations with girlfriends did happen, but not on a group scale.

In those years we were ratting and spraying our hair, and my high school yearbook photos show that literally every hair was in place. I don't know if it was me or the world at the time, but everybody else had that fakeness about them, too. Whatever I saw lacking in the mirror had mostly to do with my hair! And days could be dramatically bad, apparently, if my hair wasn't right. Heaven forbid you had a hair sticking up anywhere!

Young adulthood put me in college. I remember being on a pretty good footing; it was a good feeling not to have to worry about self-image things. I just concentrated on people, studies, and whatever else came along. I don't feel that I missed much, which is a nice feeling.

I majored in drama. I don't pretend that I am a very good actress, but I am very good in ensemble—at teamwork, as background, and as part of the cast. I don't have "star baby" qualities, but in those days I contributed solidly to the efforts of my class of thirteen in the school of drama. The experience of getting out on stage, learning to be comfortable, and allowing myself absolute stage fright was very important. There is such an adrenaline spurt in it; it's sink or swim. It is so energizing to be that nervous, that afraid, and then to be plugged into the "electricity." You go from fear to creativity. That is exciting!

College was wonderful. I started to make friends with more women because I was living with them: interesting women from totally different backgrounds, with different talents, and different interests. Cheerleading remained a thread in my life because there was no dance program at school. It was great exercise and related to drama and dance. And boys. You twirl a skirt and, hey, you have several new friends after the game.

College was very expensive. I don't know how my parents afforded it even though my mother worked. Occasionally my parents sent me a care package or a $10 bill. For increased solvency I took a job at the nearby Soldiers and Sailors Home, which was run by the Department of Children and Family Services. And I had my first look at the other side of the world—the not-so-privileged side. At the home the kids, ranging in age from preschool to high school, were wards of the state. They were not necessarily orphans: perhaps the family had thirteen children and could take care of only five. The state wrested the remaining children from the family and put them in different institutions, regardless of sibling groups. And the home then saw to their basic needs and education.

I was hired as a recreational proctor, which meant I took the kids on outings, took care of their little newsletter, stood watch while they were in recreation hall, and so on. My heart went out to these kids. One boy continually said he was going home that weekend, but it was a fantasy. Many of the girls were simply in the get-married mode. And there was little Joey who had an IQ of 69. My many experiences there led me to the concept of giving back, which I think young people need to learn. Since then I have involved myself in many projects by giving of my time and energy.

All through college, my self-image and mirror image were as high as they had ever been and I felt very secure in how I looked. Then, too, working for two years with those kids and living for one year at the home, I began to set adult priorities that didn't include "How do I look?" How could looks be important? These children had so little that the most important thing to them was their name; it was the only thing they owned. I listened to them and remembered their names—a simple thing, but it meant that the kids would gravitate toward me, which the home didn't like. I was constantly reprimanded in the headmaster's office for getting too friendly with the children or for touching them. But I remember vividly how they responded to a kind touch of the hand.

One time I was asked to take a van-load of ten kids to the TeenFair at Navy Pier in Chicago. The home gave them $1.50 apiece for the day in Chicago! Well, it was gone like that, and because I had very little money in my own pocket, when it was time to go home the kids hadn't had a meal. So I rang up my folks, who lived in the direction of the home, and said, "I've got ten kids and no food!" So the kids were invited to meet my parents, see my room, and have dinner and brownies. It was so obvious that these kids had had no role models—the absolute building blocks of life. Just to go to somebody's home and have dinner was an event in their lives. How to operate in a family was a mystery to them.

On the way home from my folks' house the conversation was all about what my life was like! Then I became aware that even if you play a teeny part in someone's life, you still have an impact because you influence other souls as you go. You can't be insular and not give back to them. That was a terrific experience and yet so frustrating.

After graduation, I taught high school: a fast-track English class, one for average kids, and two classes of nonreading juniors. Those non-readers had no tools and yet I learned so much from them. One class was composed of 21 big and burly boys. I was an idealistic new teacher and had been advised to just babysit for them. They weren't mainstreamed or even issued textbooks. Once in school they were sent to study hall with lots of time on their hands. By the time I got them, their energy level was non-existent, so I taught them how to fill out job applications and various forms from the post office.

Without language skills, these kids had less ability to function in day-to-day ways. They were not without common sense knowledge, but if they couldn't read, they became isolated. How could they understand instructions? How could they better themselves? That was a very valuable lesson to me. I became acutely aware of the skills I have, which I never want to lose.

The single most important thing I have done as an adult to establish my self-image is to solidify my relationship with God. My spirituality is a solid base that allows me to have freedom and joy because I feel so solidly rooted. And it is the same with my self-image. I may be having a good mirror day or a bad one, but my base is secure and my husband is also very supportive, very loving, and nurturing. Once I have this kind of freedom, appearances pale by comparison. Not that I ignore appearance;

it's always been important to feel that I look good to go out in the world, but it has ceased to be a dominant thing. I know I have more to offer.

My appearance, personality, intellect and achievements are all very integrated. I think that as you get more comfortable with yourself as a whole, your looks become less important because you get caught up in the momentum of how you feel about yourself. As you get older, even if it's evident, being current-looking and natural-looking makes you better than ever. And the momentum of life experience fuels your self esteem.

How do I plan to deal with aging? My best clue to that is my husband because he's 76. I take my cues from him. He likes to be part of the now, to see what's happening and to join in. He sees change as stimulating— even death and things that don't seem positive—because everything has momentum, and if you don't allow yourself to change, new things will never happen. The challenge is for all of us to fit in to every age and every change that comes along in life.

Making female friends has been so enriching. I am so impressed with women. I think women should do and be whatever they possibly can and it's such fun to discover that being with your own sex is as important as being with the opposite sex. It is good for women to solidify that concept.

Women often don't get enough feedback from others about how they are perceived. If the women's movement could do any one thing, it would be to ensure that employers give women good, valuable feedback. It's been my experience that most women are taught to "settle for." That's no good. They could be happier along the way if people helped them build a better self-image. There have always been people in my life who were secure enough in themselves to compliment me or nurture me. And that's what parenting, religion, and even good jobs should be about: nurturing. I love that word. Everyone thrives on it. If you asked most people about their favorite teacher or best job, they would probably tell you about someone who took an interest in them.

I am not a media basher, but I think as women we fall prey to the media concepts of thinness and blondness. If we could teach women anything it would be how to pick and choose what works for them. As little girls we learn to feel we have to be something we are not. And a lot of women take that burden on themselves as a requirement. It's just monstrous.

There are times when I can't help noticing how conscious other women are of themselves and others. They are living a very hard life because it's a burden to always have to look perfect. I feel that if someone is perfectionistic about her appearance, she is probably overcompensating for something else.

Conversely, it's tough to say that I really don't care about my appearance. Because of my drama background, I see life as a series of vignettes, so if I were driven by any appearance motive, it would be to look special at certain times. I have always loved costumes, so getting dressed up for a special occasion is fun. If it's a gala, I love to look special. I'm happy when it all comes together, but I've also been lucky that I could always do my own hair. Which reminds me of a story.

I was in a beauty salon when a woman came in who looked just perfect. I said to the stylist, "Gee, she looks just terrific!" And the stylist said, "She should! She comes here three times a day to have her hair combed!" Well, that was a time issue I simply couldn't grasp. This was just to have her hair combed! And if she had it combed three times a day, how many days did she devote to having it washed and styled?

TUCKER, 26:
multicultural consultant

As a child I was always conscious of having one of the darkest skin shades in my family. My grandmother is very, very light-skinned with freckles; my mother has caramel skin. Skin shade had never been a family issue; however, when I got to school I learned that it mattered somehow, and that confused me. The idea that I was really dark stuck with me for a long time: I wouldn't swim or go in the sun. I'm not really sure when I first became aware of that issue, but that's the clearest memory I have of my appearance.

I grew up with my mother and grandmother. My grandmother had seven sisters who were living when I was a child; two of them were twins who lived upstairs in the same building and often babysat for me. I remember clearly that whenever I went to someone's house it was a great affair. I was, and still am, made to feel very special within the family. That contributes to who I am and my feeling that everyone should be happy to see me. It sounds conceited but it does a lot for my self-image, especially on those days when I am not so happy to be wherever I am.

For the first seven years of my life I was an only girl-child with all those aunties. I was exposed to a lot of things. I was treated like an adult. I sat on a kitchen step stool and watched them cook; I asked questions and listened to stories about their work as domestics for very rich families. As the other children came along, we were all very much appreciated. Along with that, my grandmother very consciously encouraged all of us to do, and be, and have the things we wanted. Whatever we showed interest in, she proclaimed great. And that applied equally to the boys as well as the girls.

My mother always put my artwork up on the refrigerator regardless of its merit; dancing school recitals were a great affair and the whole family had to go, even though I wasn't much of a ballerina. I appreciate all that now. I am the oldest, and also the first granddaughter, so that may account for some of the hoopla. It wasn't that I was so pretty as a child, but I had a lot of positive energy. There wasn't a focus on my looks or my clothes, but lots of attention was showered on me.

My mother, who worked in a management position at a large corporation, has been married three times. When I was 8 she divorced her second husband, so between ages 8 and 14 I lived with my mother and my little brother. That affected who I am, too, especially my sense of independence. My mother spent lots of time with us. She didn't necessarily push us but she wanted us to try things: baseball, softball, bowling, dancing school, and clay modeling.

When I was 14, she got married again and we moved from a large midwestern city to a small town of 33,000 people, where we lived with my new stepdad and his five children. That was a major turning point in my life. I hated the town and everyone in it. Initially I didn't get along with my stepsiblings at all. They were jealous of me; they thought I had everything and that I was spoiled. As a result, I spent those high school years very detached from my family and that town. The high school environment was very regimented: everyone had to act the same, look the same, wear the same things. Being from the city, I hated the conformity: it was boring and artificially imposed upon us. It was a tough time for me.

As a young girl who was bigger and taller than my classmates, I hated to go shopping for school clothes. There was nothing to wear: no sizes, no styles, even my shoe size was an eleven. I was overweight and always looked older than I was, which made it even harder to find clothes. And because all teenagers are so into the appropriate clothes, it was a disaster. In my high school, if you couldn't get the right clothes, you didn't fit in and you heard all the little comments from the other kids. Those years were terrible.

In family arguments with my new brothers and sisters, one of the issues that surfaced daily was my weight. I don't know if I thought I was overweight or if other people thought I was; I am also not sure if I really was overweight or just bigger and taller than the other kids. I have been 5' 7 1/2" inches tall since I was 13. I still feel scrutinized about my weight, even though I have learned to accept myself more.

My stepsiblings included two girls, one of whom is several years older than me, and three boys. My older stepsister and her cousin—who was initially a good friend of mine—started the hostilities. After she and I had a falling out, she began calling me "Blubber." Not just every once in a while, but constantly. That experience really stuck with me; I think it's the reason I cannot accept compliments about my appearance. I usually attribute compliments to small talk or some ulterior motive. That is problematic for me; I can't really get a measuring stick to use on myself. When people say the teenage years are tough, they're right—it all happened to me then.

When I was in high school I went through all kinds of phases trying to be different. I got haircuts, colored my hair purple, got my ear pierced five times. My appearance never elicited negatives from my parents; they allowed me to experiment. But now I see those years as a time of searching and wanting to try something other than the available options. That was my way of controlling one facet of the uncontrollable situation of the move, the new brothers and sisters, the new school, the new friends and a new household regimen. I hated being uprooted. I hated all of it. I'm still trying to get a grip on who I was; that was such a critical time for who I was, as well as for who I am now.

When my stepdad—whom I consider my dad—acknowledged that those were, in fact, hard years for everyone, I was surprised to learn that my parents had noticed. I thought I was the only one who saw our home as a crazy place. I admitted to him, however, that I wouldn't be the person I am if I had stayed in the big city. All my friends there got married young and are now mothers of three and four children. Once we moved away there was nothing else for me to do in that small town but study and practice my music. So it was really a blessing in disguise: I decided to study and go to college because I wasn't going to live forever in a place as backward as that. My goal was to get really good grades so that I could go to any school I wanted, as long as it was away from there.

I was not popular in high school; I did not even come close. Our school had lots of cliques and hierarchies. As an aspiring writer I joined a writer's workshop, which got me interacting with more students; otherwise I wouldn't have talked to anyone other than my family and the kids in the band.

I was shy and quiet, definitely not outgoing. In eighth grade I would hyperventilate when I had to get up in front of the class and give a speech. I didn't challenge people and ask questions like I do now. I wasn't as interested in my appearance, either. I was probably too insecure because of my home environment where I refrained from giving my opinion because we were all feuding. Even in undergraduate school I wasn't outgoing at all. However, I kept taking on responsibilities that required me to get up and speak in front of groups. And that is how I have gotten to where I am today: I forced myself to do the things I feared.

During my college years, I clearly remember learning what it meant to be a woman instead of a man in terms of gender and power. I had never come up against that before because my parents overcompensated with their daughters. They wanted us to be prepared to do anything: we learned to fix cars, we were encouraged to accomplish the goals we dreamed up. Once I got to college and joined a student organization, I realized that not only were all the presidents of the student organizations men, but that, as president, they were paid a salary! I couldn't understand why no one was applying for those offices, but I started campaigning.

I ran for vice president of one of the student organizations and ended up designing and implementing programs on campus, which ultimately forced me to develop a higher profile. Then I learned more about sexual politics: there were three women and four men on the board of this group and at meetings the women never got a word in edgewise! All of my really good ideas were pulled apart at the seams. Our enforced silence and ineffectiveness at those meetings is one reason why I am so outspoken these days. At that point I was still searching for my own voice; now I am putting my voice out there and I believe everyone needs to hear it! I don't feel silenced anymore. If I do, I get up and leave the situation. I no longer feel compelled to stay and work things out when I am silenced because that is the worst feeling. I need to say what I want to say and be who I want to be in groups and organizations. These days even my dad comments that I have a lot to say. So my personality and attitudes have definitely changed.

College served me well. I went to school on a journalism scholarship, which allowed me to seize a lot of leadership opportunities. My willingness grew out of the family experience: try this, try that, try everything. The result was that I grew.

When I graduated with my journalism degree, I decided to attend graduate school rather than go into journalism. As it turned out, my only choices were in New York state, which was far from my family, but I went out there all by myself and had a chance to find out more about who I really was. As someone searching, I had many opportunities to try various things before I got out into the so-called real world. I did well at most things, so I have no regrets or bad memories about those years.

I know that my perceptions of myself are totally different from other people's perceptions of me. I am still figuring that out and learning about myself. At my core, I often dismiss all the positive reinforcement, but there are people in my life who contribute constant validation. My two young half-brothers—the children of my mother's and stepfather's marriage—are very close to me. I can do no wrong in their eyes; they idolize me. They never see the imperfections that I focus on, but that's true with everyone, I guess.

My parents never had issues with my appearance and the way I carry myself. They always acted as if I could do anything. In fact, sometimes I feel a lot of pressure from my dad's high expectations. But that has been good for me, too; when I begin to doubt myself, I always know there is one person who thinks I can do anything I want to do. There are certain other people in my life who validate me no matter what. Their support is never-ending. They think I am absolutely beautiful. I may dismiss the compliment as part of their love for me, but I always know I can count on them.

Someone has suggested that I keep a journal of all the nice things people say about my appearance to help me integrate those comments into my self-perceptions. I need to focus on hearing—and believing—all the good things that people say about me, because I don't believe that I am attractive. Recently, I listed all the things I am grateful for; when I read it, I was overwhelmed. Maybe a list of compliments would do the same thing—overwhelm me with all the positive perceptions about me.

At this point in my life—even with my weight and body image issues—I am becoming more comfortable with who I am as a whole person. Knowing how standards of beauty have changed over the ages and how those standards are imposed upon us has helped. More and more, I challenge myself to hear the positive things people say or to look in the mirror and see myself as okay.

Being okay means looking at the whole color issue, too. The idea that one color is better than another is a definite imposition on people; it could just as easily be justified the other way around. One time I challenged my stepbrother on his comment about a set of twins whom he described as not very attractive. I asked him what made them unattractive; at the same time, I offered my theory that if they were three shades lighter in color, he would think they were attractive. He finally said, "You know,

I think you're right!" I have had to deprogram myself from that issue because it makes me angry. There are sororities that used to require pledges to be lighter than a brown paper bag; anyone who was a different shade had to join a different sorority. For instance, when my mother was in college, she was in one sorority and her best friend was in another. They were told they could not be friends anymore all because of the shade of their skin!

This is the first time in my life that I have positive mental images of myself. Today when I look in the mirror I love to look at my skin. That's a big change for me. I used to think that maybe I was too dark—especially when it came to dating guys in high school and college—or that my hair should be straighter, or longer, or thicker. Now I don't even think about those things. If a man felt that way about me, I wouldn't be compatible with him anyway.

Also, I now dress fabulously and I never could have said that before! Even with my current weight and my size eleven shoes, I look great all the time. At one time I worked at Lane Bryant and thought I had to have all kinds of clothes, but I don't even do that anymore. I feel great about the way I put myself together. I am just hitting my stride these days and I really look better than ever. My most positive mental image of myself includes that of a strong woman with a real presence and an inner light.

The whole idea of loving self is something I am only beginning to believe in. Three years ago I would have said that I loved myself, but I don't really feel that I was coming into my own the way I am now. I really look forward to what's ahead: baggage to leave behind and things to learn. All this self-knowledge feeds directly into my belief that I look better than ever.

The writer bell hooks talks about how women scrutinize themselves in the mirror and always find fault. So for a long time I have worked at appreciating my reflection: I look in the mirror every morning and tell myself I am beautiful. As a teenager I remember looking at myself naked in the bathroom mirror—I had read that women should do that to appreciate their bodies—but I had a completely negative reaction. There were times in my younger years when I would not even wear shorts or a swimsuit. I probably weigh more now than I did then, but I no longer have that same response, even though I think I need to lose weight and get in shape. This past summer I wore a swimsuit at the beach. So that baggage is diminished, although not completely gone.

The first time anyone ever told me I was beautiful, my reaction was, "Did he mean that?" For the most part, when people talk about their perceptions of me, they don't talk about my physical appearance; they talk about my presence or approachability. I know I don't accept compliments well, and I really want to turn that situation around. I realize that it's not always easy for men to give out compliments, either. They must want them to be received well or they wouldn't offer them

I am now on an eating-well program and have started working out. The woman who inspired me to work out told me that I would look in the mirror for the longest time without registering a change in my image in my own head. And she was right. Although I have joined a health club and am going regularly, I haven't really accepted a new image of me as having lost weight. However, I am amazed at what a difference exercise can make. I hated to exercise until this past summer; now I love it. I love the way my body changed. I want to keep exercising and see what happens.

I have no idea how I will deal with the aging process. There is one thing I am blessed with: all my life there have been older women role models for me. My grandma and her sisters were all beautiful women and I saw that very clearly, so aging is not a big negative: it's what success is. I look forward to that sense of success. Those women were the center of our universe when we were kids, and my mom's generation was the extension of that center.

As women we have so few opportunities to talk about all these issues that we can't even unload them, much less figure out how to deal with them. Although I keep a journal, I have not written about these past issues to any extent; I usually deal very much with the present. I never thought much about the disparity between mirror image and internalized self-image, which comes from all the baggage we bring with us from the beginning of our lives. I forget that there is a long history behind why I feel the way I do about myself. It's very exciting to begin to put these things into perspective!

FROM A
TINY SEED

It has been said that if you are meant to accomplish a project, you will grow into the person capable of executing that project. I have certainly grown with this project over the past ten years. It has taken on a life of its own, taken over most of my life, and has begun to blossom more exuberantly than my faithful and treasured coffee-table African violet.

If, ten years ago, I wondered where my life and energies were headed I no longer wonder. If I wondered why my past appeared to be full of so many seemingly disparate experiences, I no longer wonder. Once the seeds of this book project were sown, it literally took root, generating itself. As its first tiny shoots appeared and its growth and development proved to be irresistible, I found all my life experiences coming to bear on it, as well as, coming into flower upon it.

The original idea for the book germinated with a suggestion from a consultant-to-budding-authors whom I met at a small business seminar. She suggested I write a book about professional wardrobing to help promote my image consulting business. However, once the concept sprouted, it quickly went beyond her idea for a simple image book and converged with my impulse to do something more meaningful around the psychological issues of women's appearance. Once I decided to interview women about their lived experience of appearance, the project had a format. Once I started listening to, empathizing with, and taping the stories, the project began to unfold with the voluptuous urgency of flora reaching toward the sunshine.

Soon afterward, at a seminar on realizing your dream, I learned that if you tell everyone you meet about your dream, they will help you make it come true! And that is exactly what has happened. Once I initiated the interviewing process, there began to appear a steady and seemingly never-ending flow of people who nourished and fertilized and tended to the needs of the book-in-the-making. The list of these associate dream-makers and the stories of their support, enthusiasm, concern, advice, networking, and volunteerism would fill another volume.

While more and more women presented themselves to me with amazing stories to tell, my husband kept the computer running. One day, an unsuspecting yet empathic free-lance editor walked through the door of my office. She initially directed me toward books on how to find literary agents and publishers. She later edited the entire manuscript. Several self-published authors crossed my path and shared their experiences. Then articles started showing up in magazines describing the new technologies of print-on-demand books and electronic publishing. Self-publishing became a viable option when I met a woman who runs a desk-top publishing business. She arranged the design and production of the book and solved the problem of where to store it and how to ship it.

Along the way, my often-dreamed-of opportunity to attend graduate school, while further pursuing women's issues, suddenly became a reality. Several years into both the project and my graduate studies, a high-school friend telephoned long distance. She was organizing a women's conference at the small liberal arts college where she worked, and she generously invited me to present some of my interview material on body image. As a result of this presentation, one of the associate professors at the college showed interest in the manuscript as a potential text for her women's studies course and, in doing so, redefined its potential scope.

As the interviews became a manuscript and the manuscript became a set of galleys, other issues needed to be addressed. Many friends have read chapters and given feedback. When some aspects of entertainment law needed to be researched, a friend who had just finished law school and passed the bar, agreed to look into such matters. When I remembered a piece of artwork, seen years ago, that I thought would be perfect for the book cover, another friend told me how to go about getting the rights to it.

When it came time to think about promoting the book and the internet seemed like a logical place to start, the desk-top publisher supplied a web-site designer. When it came time to think about publicizing the book, a strategy-savvy friend with her own public relations business reappeared on the scene. And when it came time to think about marketing the book, one friend after another offered suggestions and potential orders: one friend, who buys books and gifts for a home-town retail store, is interested in the book and an author's reading; several other friends have requested the book, along with an author's reading, for their book club. And so the project grows and grows.

If it is true, therefore, that I have grown into the person capable of accomplishing the book project of my dreams, it is equally true that the metamorphosis of myself and the project has not taken place without the considerable and sustaining momentum of my associate dream-makers. It is also true that the project has grown into a living organism, a flowering plant like my African violet. It continually puts forth fresh blooms in the form of creative offshoots which, in turn, generate new enthusiasms and new directions. There seems to be no limit to the growth potential for both myself and my appearances project.

OCTOBER 31, 2000

S P E A K I N G   O U T

Although several of the stories in this book describe the interviewee's experience of reconstructive and/or cosmetic surgery as a part of her search for an improved appearance and self-image, this book is in no way intended as a vehicle to promote said surgery and should not be considered as such. Neither the book nor the author take any position other than a neutral one which affirms and values each woman's right to choose such surgery or to refrain from it. Neither the book nor the author are in any way connected with any person or organization which promotes or performs reconstructive or cosmetic surgery. The use of this book for any such promotional purpose would constitute misuse.

One of the main reasons for undertaking this book of interviews was to educate myself in the ways that other women have dealt with the lived experience of their appearance. I have since learned much about the universal difficulties of being a woman in our culture and have developed a much greater sense of my uniqueness as well as my membership in the community of women.

It would have been so helpful if, during the terrible teen years, my friends and I had been able to discuss these issues openly. Unfortunately, we were well into our thirties before we started to admit our youthful angst to each other: "I thought I was the only one who felt that way!" we sighed and then laughed. Now we talk about anything and everything, hoping to help each other through either the current crisis or the current triumph.

It has not been easy to get past my ambivalence about putting my own story into print. Others felt the experience of talking about selfhood was very therapeutic. In fact, a therapist-friend enthusiastically encouraged the project as an important forum for women's voices to be heard by other women in discussion of female issues of appearance. Providing that forum, then, has been an equally important reason for undertaking as well as finishing this book. It has been a long time in the process, but as the manuscript moves beyond a work-in-progress to become an actual book, the voices may now be heard. The words may now be read. The stories may now be shared.

The Importance
of Stories

God created man because He loved the stories.
THE TALMUD

I need not feel isolated if I know that there are
other comrades with similar experiences.
bell hooks

Coming to selfhood...cannot happen in isolation.
bell hooks

I have to tell stories to go on living
and to change the world.
DOROTHY ALLISON

Most people resonate more to the stories than to
the psychological tests and statistical results.
JASON BRANDT

THEMES AND ISSUES FOR DISCUSSION

Acting

Aging

Ambivalence

Anorexia

Art

Athletic ability; lack of

Appropriate female behavior

Assertiveness: innate; learned

Attitude, outlook

Balance

Beautiful mothers, sisters

Being well behaved, considerate

Braces

Bone structure

Bulimia

Challenging behavior

Creativity

Clothes we loved; clothes
we hated

Comparisons to others

Competitiveness

Compliments; lack of;
constraints against

Controlling parents

Corrective surgery

Dance

Diets, dieting

Disruptive behavior

Dyslexia

Education

Eyes, vision

Enhancing your looks

Expectations of female
appearance and behavior:
cultural; familial; peer group;
self-imposed

Fashion

Fashion design

Feeling good about ourselves

Feet

Femaleness

Femininity

Femininization

Glasses

Growth spurts

Hair, bad/good; hair color;
hairstyles

Height

Health

Illness

Inappropriate treatment from
others

Insults; insensitive remarks

Intelligence

Interests, skills, accomplishments

Intimidating behavior

Jealousy

Kinesthesia

Leadership

Lesbianism

Life experience

Lifestyle

Looking just like your
mother/father

Makeup, cosmetics

Male attitudes toward females

Maturation: early; late

Media, advertising

Mixed messages

Mother's taste in clothes vs.
  daughter's taste

Music

Negative feedback; lack of

Nicknames

Nose

Nutrition

Oppressive imagery

Parents: competitive; difficult;
  embarrassing; supportive

Personal growth and development

Personality

Physical limitations

Pleasing others

Pregnancy

Pressure: cultural; peer; familial

Pretty and smart

Professional image

Positive feedback; lack of

Popularity

Purposefulness

Purpose in life

Resemblance to other family
  members; lack of

Role models

Rocking the boat!

Sewing

Sex appeal

Self-consciousness

Shaming by parents; teachers

Shyness

Sibling friendships, respect

Sibling insults

Sibling rivalry

Skin color

Smart and pretty

Smile, personality projection

Smile, self-conscious

Smile, make nice

Sports

Squelching of enthusiasm;
  inquisitiveness; talkativeness;
  assertiveness; adventurousness

Struggle for individuality

Supportive relatives and
  adult friends

Supposed to be a boy

Teen icons of beauty

Teeth

Tomboyishness

Unwanted sexual attention

Values regarding appearance

Vocal quality

"Voice"

Weight

Wrinkles